A PRIMER ON LYMPHEDEMA

Deborah G. Kelly, PT, MSEd

Associate Professor of Physical Therapy
University of Kentucky

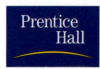
Prentice Hall

Upper Saddle River, New Jersey 07458

Library of Congress Cataloging-in-Publication Data

Kelly, Deborah G.
    A primer on lymphedema / Deborah G. Kelly.
      p. ; cm.
    Includes bibliographical references and index.
    ISBN 0-13-022410-3
    1. Lymphedema. I. Title.
    [DNLM: 1. Lymphedema—therapy. 2. Lymphatic System—physiology. 3.
    Lymphedema—diagnosis. WH 700 K298p 2002]
    RC646.3 K45 2002
    616.4'2—dc21   2001036676

Publisher: Julie Levin Alexander
Senior Acquisitions Editor: Mark Cohen
Assistant Editor: Melissa Kerian
Managing Editor: Patrick Walsh
Production Management: bookworks
Production Editor: Lisa Garboski
Director of Production and Manufacturing : Bruce Johnson
Manufacturing Manager: Ilene Sanford
Creative Director: Cheryl Asherman
Design Coordinator: Maria Guglielmo-Walsh
Composition: Peirce Graphic Services
Marketing Manager: David Hough
Product Information Manager: Rachele Triano
Printer/Binder: RR Donnelley & Sons, Crawfordsville, IN
Copy Editor: Patricia Wilson
Proofreader: Wayne Beatty
Cover Design: Blair Brown
Cover Illustration: HUMAN ANATOMY 3/E by Martini/Timmons/McKinley,© 2000. Reprinted by permission of Pearson Education, Inc., Upper Saddle River, NJ.
Cover Printer: Phoenix Color Corporation

Notice: The author and the publisher of this volume have taken care that the information and technical recommendations contained herein are based on research and expert consultation, and are accurate and compatible with the standards generally accepted at the time of publication. Nevertheless, as new information becomes available, changes in clinical and technical practices become necessary. The reader is advised to carefully consult manufacturers' instructions and information material for all supplies and equipment before use, and to consult with a health care professional as necessary. This advice is especially important when using new supplies or equipment for clinical purposes. The author and publisher disclaim all responsibility for any liability, loss, injury, or damage incurred as a consequence, directly or indirectly, of the use and application of any of the contents of this volume.

Pearson Education LTD.
Pearson Education Australia PTY, Limited
Pearson Education Singapore, Pte. Ltd
Pearson Education North Asia Ltd
Pearson Education Canada, Ltd.
Pearson Educación de Mexico, S.A. de C.V.
Pearson Education — Japan
Pearson Education Malaysia, Pte. Ltd.

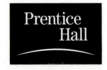

10 9 8 7 6 5 4 3 2 1
ISBN 0-13-022410-3

CONTENTS

PREFACE

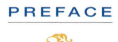

In recent years, health professionals in North America have devoted increased attention to patients with lymphedema and the treatment options available to them. The condition itself is not new. The signs and symptoms have existed but have been largely ignored or ineffectively treated for decades. With the significant incidence of lymphedema in North America and around the world, there is a clamor from patients and health professionals for more information, improved education, and increased access to effective treatment methods. Successful treatment options from Europe and Australia have attracted considerable interest since no prior method has been satisfactory in managing the symptoms over time.

In part because of improvements in health care delivery, the number of patients seeking treatment for lymphedema is significant. Statistics convey a wide range on the rate of incidence.[1] Some have speculated that lymphedema will become more prevalent over time. Reasons for the size of this patient population include:

- Improved survivorship following cancer treatment has allowed patients to live long enough to develop the symptoms, which can appear many years after surgery or other cancer treatment.
- Aggressive sampling and dissection of lymph nodes for various types of cancer treatment, although on the decline, has been the accepted norm for many years.
- Debilitating effects of radiation therapy are reduced now with more specific treatments, but like other systems in the body, the long-term effects to the lymphatic system may continue to surface for another decade before they begin to decline.
- Incidence of certain types of cancers, such as melanoma and prostate, and subsequent treatment is still rising.
- Assertiveness and awareness of patients seeking care contributes to the number of people identified with lymphedema.
- Slow but steady improvement among practitioners in the recognition and accurate diagnosis of lymphedema has increased the number of individuals recognized with the signs and symptoms.
- Access to the Internet has raised consciousness about the signs and symptoms of lymphedema, leading to improved detection.

As this patient population looks to the medical community for a response, professionals are seeking the most current information and education to return this group

---

[1]Refer to Chapter 2 for an extensive list of citations on incidence of lymphedema in various populations.

back to functional and normal, or near normal, lives. Currently, referring practitioners do not designate what level of education a clinician must have before treating a patient with lymphedema. It can be assumed, therefore, that new graduates as well as experienced clinicians are faced with the challenge of how to treat the signs and symptoms of this diagnosis and when to refer on to a specially educated clinician. As cited throughout this text, individuals with lymphedema must have their symptoms managed appropriately from their onset to minimize the sequelae. Symptoms usually become more profound with time. While intervention at any time in the disease process can lead to improvements, the most significant and lasting gains are seen when appropriate intervention is initiated as soon as signs and symptoms appear.

This is an exciting time for people interested in lymphedema and management of the symptoms. There are articles, now numbering in the thousands, that contribute to the information explosion on the lymphatic system. Many issues are on the table for discussion among medical professionals: scientific merit of current treatments, efficacy of treatment, adherence behaviors, measures of quality of life, patient satisfaction, clinical outcomes, certification, scope of practice, payment, use of alternative medical therapies, use of alternative compression devices, the paradigm shift in historical treatments, and the use of dietary, pharmaceutical, and surgical intervention as adjunct therapy. Watch the literature closely over the next few years for information on these topics. There is still much to learn about these and other issues. Among the most promising projects are investigations that may lead to possible breakthroughs in the use of gene therapy to de-bulk tumors, and the use of techniques for autotransplant of lymphocytes into lymphedematous limbs to reduce the symptoms of lymphedema.

My primary goal in writing this text is to provide an enticing, readable, visually informative resource for health professionals and students in professional programs. This text is unique in that it will serve many needs for a variety of health professions. The text will facilitate clinical decision-making and will provide information for in-service presentations, provider relations meetings, communications with referral sources, intervention plans, and clinical specialization.

Special elements are included in the text to enhance the learning experience for practitioners and students alike: excellent anatomical illustrations, color photos of actual patients, case studies, graphs, educational handouts to be copied, current references, and quotes from leaders in the field. The value and the venue of this book is broad so that buyers may purchase it to expand their knowledge of the lymphatic system, but could also use it to improve their documentation skills, and increase their understanding of current issues such as reimbursement and the disablement model of patient/client management. I have written with the mind of an educator, the heart of a clinician, and the will of an activist. It is my hope that readers will aspire to at least one of these roles by the end of this text.

ACKNOWLEDGMENTS

When I think of the experts around the world who have put their professional energy, research efforts, and countless clinical hours into the topic of lymphedema, I am humbled to be a part of that process. I am fortunate to be able to follow my passion and share it with others. Writing a book would have been a very lonely endeavor without the support of many people. I gratefully acknowledge these people and their contributions:

- Mark Cohen, Prentice Hall Acquisitions editor, who began this project with me. He was exceedingly supportive even with my frequently used comment: "I should have no trouble meeting that deadline." Special thanks to Patrick Walsh, Lisa Garboski, and all the members of the Prentice Hall team who brought this edition to completion so efficiently.
- Günter Klose, a gifted instructor, an inspiration to all who know him, generous beyond measure with his time and talents.
- The physical therapy faculty at the University of Kentucky. Thank you for your encouragement, friendship, editorial comments, and valuable insights. There isn't a better faculty cohort to work alongside anywhere.
- Our division staff assistants who gave me consistent staff support to keep my other academic commitments running smoothly during this project.
- Clinical colleagues from our original Lymphedema Management team at the University of Kentucky Clinic. Our team meetings, program building, and patient care experiences have been fodder for the book. You are true partners, supporting my enthusiasm yet tempering it with reality.
- The contributors who participated in the book. Your contributions added visual and practical interest, and broadened the venue of the text. Special thanks to Janice Kuperstein, Barbara Ann Murphy, Carrie Sullivan, Maureen Fleagle, Günter Klose, and Steve Norton.
- Student reviewers Sarah Harvieux SPT-Class of 2002 and Ashley Buren OTS-Class of 2001, who took time from their busy lives to reflect critically on the text from a student perspective.
- The physical therapy students from the University of Kentucky who have expressed interest in the project and concern for my progress semester after semester during which my endless litany was "It's coming along . . ."
- The many courageous patients who contributed through their comments, photographs, and efforts in therapy to achieve a healthier, more normal life.
- Most important, the members of my family:
    My parents, who read Chapter 1 a few years ago and never let on that I had a long way to go. My daughters Shannon and Faryn, your love notes, and patient understanding made it possible to continue. My husband Bob, helper,

confidant, and unwitting research assistant. You have been the encourager supreme even in the midst of your own research. This project would not have happened without your love and support.

The publisher and the author gratefully acknowledge the following reviewers, whose comments and suggestions contributed to the quality of this text.

Sharon Potter Anderson, PT, DrPH
Associate Professor
Department of Physical Therapy
Loma Linda University
Loma Linda, California

Pamela D. Ritzline, PT, MS
Director and Assistant Professor
Physical Therapist Assistant Program
University of Indianapolis
Krannert School of Physical Therapy
Indianapolis, Indiana

PART I

UNDERSTANDING LYMPHEDEMA

A growing body of information on how the lymphatic system functions has changed the way intervention is planned. In addition to new techniques, there are a variety of historical treatments still in use. Before delivery of any intervention, planning decisions should be based on appropriate knowledge of the anatomic and physiologic principles of the lymphatic system.

More than five decades of research on the lymphatic system have established the knowledge base appreciated today. The rate and level of scientific inquiry has increased rapidly in the last 10 years, making these exciting times to be examining this fascinating circulatory system. The use of lymphography has given current knowledge about lymphedema a sound morphological foundation. Large lymph vessels and lymph nodes have become accessible to direct observation. Landmark publications have focused on the function of the initial lymphatic pathways, tissue homeostasis, and the role played by the microlymphatics in the drainage of fluid from the interstitium. The techniques of flourescence microlymphography and indirect lymphography have been used to demonstrate the vessels of the initial lymphatic pathways. These techniques allow the superficial lymph capillary networks of the skin to be seen under a microscope. Permeability of lymph capillaries and flow velocity can also be evaluated.

A fresh look at the lymphatic system and its role in fluid management should entice the experienced anatomist and the curious student to further examine this complex circulatory system, which has yet to be completely understood.

Defining lymphedema will include dividing the condition into primary and secondary types and discussing current thought on etiology and predictors of onset. Clinical diagnosis is usually made without invasive tests. Occasionally more sophisticated and invasive tests are indicated, which will be described.

Managing the patient/client with lymphedema is a multifaceted task requiring skill and expertise. Part 1 of this text will conclude by taking the reader through the steps in the initial patient–therapist relationship and the examination process. Current and anticipated changes in the patient/client management model and a suggested documentation template will serve as a useful guide toward a comprehensive approach to intervention.

1

ANATOMY AND PHYSIOLOGY OF THE LYMPHATIC SYSTEM WITH CLINICAL IMPLICATIONS

" . . . thirty years ago one of the first lymph researchers in the United States . . . prophesized that the lymph system would be recognized as the most important organic system in humans and animals."

DR. EMIL VODDER (1978)

INTRODUCTION

All medical professionals have studied the role of the lymphatic system in resisting illness in the human body. Yet, the system has another essential role that it fulfills: fluid management. More specifically, fluid management refers to the life-essential role of maintaining normal microlymphatic homeostasis. A more detailed look into the function of the system and the characteristics of its primary components is not only interesting but imperative for a clear understanding of what occurs in the normal and abnormal lymph system, and for determining why certain clinical interventions may be successful while others are not. With this knowledge, health professionals can apply current clinical intervention with the assurance that anatomical and physiological principles have been respected.

I. **Function**

   The lymphatic system has two primary functions:

   A. Protect the body from infection and disease via the immune response: production, maintenance, and distribution of lymphocytes.

   B. Facilitate fluid movement from the tissues back into the bloodstream. This fluid transport will maintain normal blood volume and eliminate chemical imbalances in the interstitial fluid.

   An excellent summary of the functions of the lymphatic system can be found in the text by Martini.[1]

II. **Primary components and their characteristics**

   The lymphatic system is not a continuous set of tubes as was imagined before the electron microscope and isotopic lymphography illumined the complex and remarkable way in which the human body is equipped to move lymphatic fluid. The components of the lymphatic system are:

   • Lymphatic vessels: superficial, intermediate, and deep
   • Lymph fluid

FIGURE 1-1 Lymphatic System

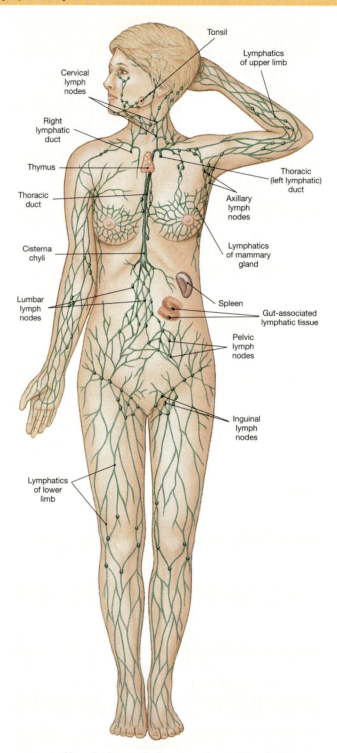

An overview of the arrangement of lymphatic vessels, lymph nodes, and lymphoid organs.

(Courtesy of *Human Anatomy, 3/e* by Martini/Timmons/McKinley© 2000. Reprinted by permission of Pearson Education, Inc., Upper Saddle River, NJ.)

- Lymph tissues and organs (including lymph nodes)
- Thoracic duct, right lymphatic duct, and lymphovenous anastomoses

A. **Lymphatic vessels** are also referred to in the literature as *lymphatics*. They are responsible for the absorption, collection, and transport of lymph throughout the body.

   1. The process begins with the smallest and most peripheral of the lymphatics, referred to as the *initial lymphatics, terminal lymphatics, superficial lymphatics,* or *lymphatic capillaries*. These initial lymphatics are found in the subcutaneous layer beneath the skin as well as in mucous membrane linings of various body tracts.[1] They are located in almost all tissues and organs of the body with the exception of the CNS and the cornea. Their structure is similar to a venous blood capillary with a few important differences. Probably the most important difference is the presence of (relatively) large openings between cell junctions in the capillary. The openings between cells allow fluids and large solutes such as protein molecules to enter the capillary. The overlapping design of the endothelial cell junction creates a one-way valve, however, so that the fluids and large solutes cannot flow back out. Opening of the *flaps* or *overlaps* is stimulated by several mechanisms including variations in tissue pressure (discussed in the next section) and contraction of *fibrils* or *anchoring filaments* attached to the exterior cell walls and surrounding connective tissue. The effects of pressure changes on the opening of cell junctions are understood; however, investigators are still gathering information about what stimulates the fibrils to contract and move the cell flaps into the open position. An increase in interstitial fluid will cause a pull on the fibrils, which will open the flaps. External, mechanical stimulation to superficial connective tissue, such as gentle skin tractioning, may contribute to flap opening by pulling on the anchoring filaments.[2]

   2. Lymphatic capillaries empty fluid into larger vessels called *precollectors,* which have the absorbing qualities of the smaller capillaries and the transporting qualities of the larger vessels. The pre-collectors are identified as intermediate vessels, which signify a change in form and function.[3] As vessels pass from superficial to central, cell junctions are less likely to have the flaps or opening feature, and walls become thicker and less permeable to large molecules. Valves are also evident in the precollectors. Precollectors expedite fluid movement from the superficial, absorptive capillaries to the deeper, transport vessels.

   3. Larger lymphatic vessels are called *collectors, lymphatics,* or *valved vessels*. These vessels carry lymph toward the trunk, running loosely parallel to deep arteries and veins of the neck, limbs, trunk, and viscera. The collector or deep vessel walls contain contractile smooth muscle like veins but have thinner walls and valves at shorter intervals. As the vessels run deeper, the diameters grow larger. Valves are spaced closely but vary from 0.6 to 10 cm apart

FIGURE 1-2 a and b Lymphatic Capillaries

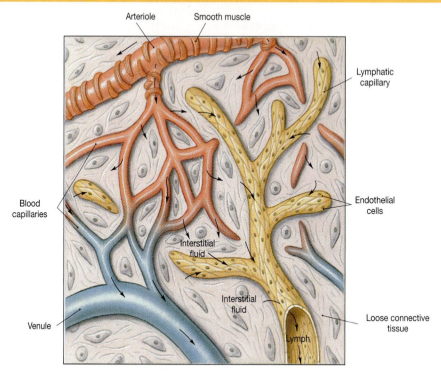

Arteriole   Smooth muscle

Lymphatic
capillary

Blood
capillaries

Endothelial
cells

Interstitial
fluid

Interstitial
fluid

Loose connective
tissue

Venule

Lymph

(a) Association of blood capillaries, tissue, and lymphatic capillaries

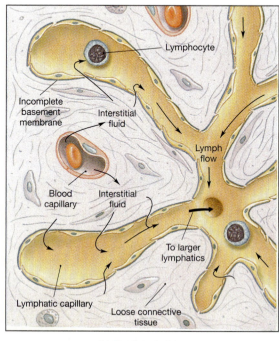

Lymphocyte

Incomplete
basement
membrane

Interstitial
fluid

Lymph
flow

Blood
capillary

Interstitial
fluid

To larger
lymphatics

Lymphatic capillary

Loose connective
tissue

(b) Sectional view

Lymphatic capillaries are blind vessels that begin in areas of loose connective tissue. **(a)** A three-dimensional view of the association of blood capillaries, tissue, interstitial fluid, and lymphatic capillaries. Interstitial fluid enters these capillaries where it now is called lymph, by passing between adjacent endothelial cells. Arrows show the direction of blood, interstitial fluid, and lymph movement. **(b)** Sectional view through a cluster of lymphatic capillaries.

(Courtesy of Prentice Hall)

(Courtesy of *Human Anatomy, 3/e* by Martini/Timmons/McKinley© 2000. Reprinted by permission of Pearson Education, Inc., Upper Saddle River, N.J.)

FIGURE 1-3 a, b, c Lymphatic Vessels and Valves

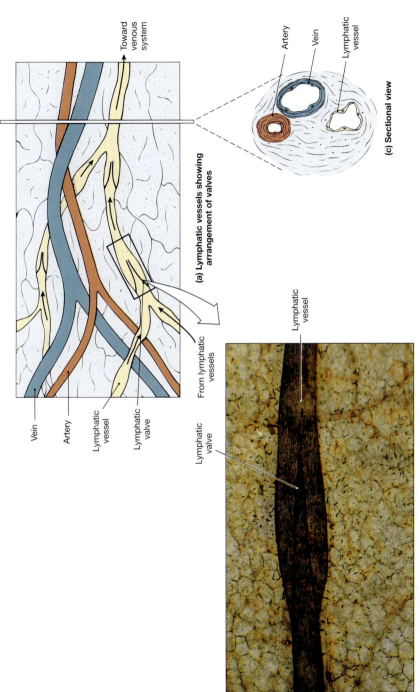

(a) Lymphatic vessels showing arrangement of valves

Toward venous system

From lymphatic vessels

Vein

Artery

Lymphatic vessel

Lymphatic valve

Artery

Vein

Lymphatic vessel

(c) Sectional view

Lymphatic valve

Lymphatic vessel

(b) Whole mount of lymphatic vessel with valve

Valves in lymphatic vessels prevent backflow of lymph. **(a)** A diagrammatic view of loose connective tissue, showing small blood vessels and a lymphatic vessel. Arrows indicate the direction of lymph flow. **(b)** Whole mount of lymphatic vessel. Lymphatic valves resemble those of the venous system. Each valve consists of a pair of flaps that permit fluid movement in only one direction. **(c)** The cross-sectional view emphasizes the structural differences between blood vessels and lymphatic vessels.

(Courtesy of *Human Anatomy, 3/e* by Martini/Timmons/McKinley© 2000. Reprinted by permission of Pearson Education, Inc., Upper Saddle River, NJ.)

7

based on the diameter of the vessel. How the valves function to move lymph will be discussed in the next section on lymph circulation. For more in-depth study of the lymph vessels refer to a current anatomy and physiology text.

Clinical Implications: Intervention for edema and lymphedema should begin with attention and care given to the superficial, initial lymphatics. The initial lymphatics are often overlooked when intervention is planned. Many historical treatments have proven to be too aggressive and have caused complications to the recovery process. If vessels are occluded by heavy pressures, absorption will be slowed or stopped. Examples of potentially heavy pressures are numerous and range from deep massage to tight clothing. Temperature, in addition to pressure, will alter capillary activity. If superficial temperature changes are extreme, capillaries will react with local hyperemia, bringing more water and subsequently more edema to the area. Examples of superficial temperature changes also vary but include application of heat or cold modalities. In the individual with a normal lymphatic system, the same capillary reactions are seen. A normal lymphatic system, however, is able to recover or accommodate for temporary insults (albeit slowly) to the superficial capillaries. Those with lymphedema or even a "limb at risk" may experience marked exacerbation of symptoms due to inappropriate amounts of pressure, heat, or cold.

B. **Lymph fluid** resembles plasma but under normal conditions contains a lower concentration of protein. After interstitial fluid enters the initial lymph capillaries the fluid is called lymph. The principal contents of the fluid called lymph are:

1. *Protein molecules:* Under normal conditions approximately half of the protein molecules in circulation will be transported by the lymphatic system from the interstitium back to the systemic circulation in a period of one day.

2. *Water:* Water serves as a transport medium for the cellular products being moved toward the venous system.

3. *Cellular components:* Numerous and diverse, cellular content of the fluid will include white blood cells, cancer cells, bacterial and viral cells, and cellular debris from proteolysis and phagocytosis.

4. *Fatty acids:* Certain lipids absorbed by the intestinal tract will travel via the lymphatic vessels to reach the bloodstream.

Clinical Implications: When the lymphatic system is unable to keep up with the demands of fluid overload for any reason, lymph will become protein-rich and at the same time stagnant. This environment creates an ideal culture for the growth of pathogens, increasing the risk of infection. This risk may be present before swelling is evident. Everyone who is at risk should be educated about the signs, symptoms, and prevention of infection. Look for discussion of these issues in Chapters 2 and 4 of this text as well as a list of precautions in Chapter 8, which can be copied for patients.

C. **Lymph tissues and organs (including lymph nodes)** The distribution of lymphoid organs and tissues throughout the body is strategic. Areas

FIGURE 1-4

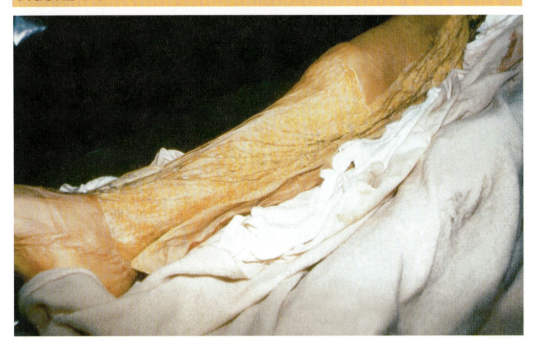

Cadaver dissection, lower extremity with deep lymphatics stained for identification.
(Courtesy of Klose Norton Training and Consulting, LLC)

of the body that are at risk of injury or pathogen invasion have a generous allocation of tissues and nodes. **Tissues** include the *tonsils* and connective tissue nodules, without fibrous capsules, in specific locations beneath epithelial linings in the body. **Organs** include the *lymph nodes, thymus,* and *spleen.* Most of the tissues and organs are designed to facilitate lymphocyte production and distribution. **Lymph nodes** are small, oval-shaped organs resembling kidney beans. They are encapsulated by dense connective tissue. Blood vessels, nerves, and lymphatic vessels attach to the body of the lymph node at specific indentations. See Figure 1.5. Lymph nodes play a role in filtering waste and in regulation of protein concentration in lymph fluid. The nodes are arranged in groups or chains. The total number of lymph nodes estimated in a typical human is 600 to 700 with about 100 to 200 of those located in the mesentery and another 160 in the neck region. The size of nodes will vary throughout the body with some being as small as 2 mm in diameter, too small or too deep to palpate. Other nodes measure up to 25 mm in diameter and are easier to identify manually. The *sentinel lymph node (SLN)* is the initial draining lymph node in a lymph region. The procedure of SLN biopsy has received much attention in recent literature for its potential to reduce the rate of complications over complete dissections (see Clinical Implications on page 11 for more details).

FIGURE 1-5 Structure of a Lymph Node

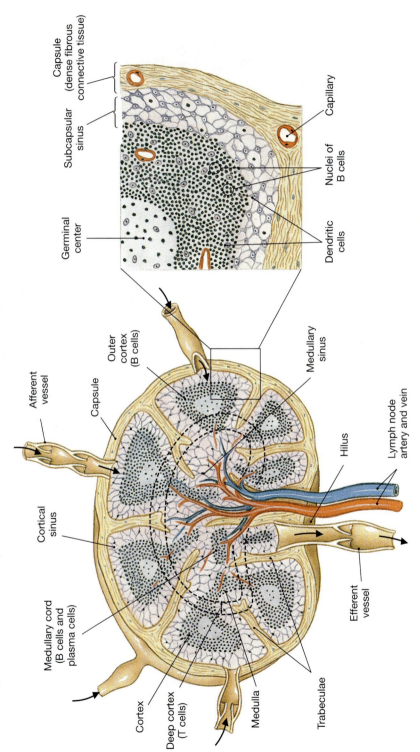

Lymph nodes are covered by a dense, fibrous, connective tissue capsule. Lymphatic vessels and blood vessels penetrate the capsule to reach the lymphoid tissue within.

(Courtesy of *Human Anatomy*, 3/e by Martini/Timmons/McKinley© 2000. Reprinted by permission of Pearson Education, Inc., Upper Saddle River, NJ.)

FIGURE 1-6 Lymphatic Drainage of the Head and Neck

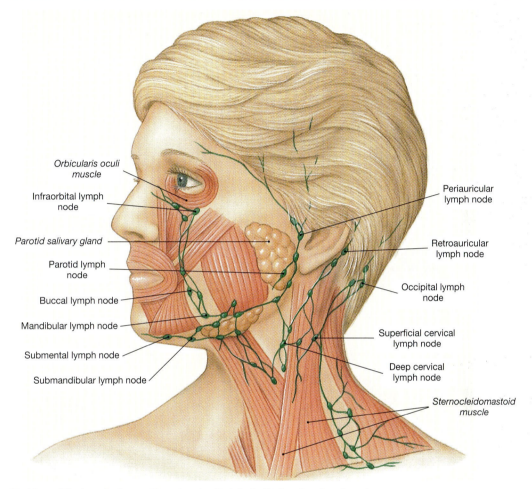

Position of the lymphatic vessels and nodes that drain the head and neck region.
(Courtesy of *Human Anatomy, 3/e* by Martini/Timmons/McKinley© 2000. Reprinted by permission of Pearson Education, Inc., Upper Saddle River, NJ.)

For more information on the complex functions of the lymph nodes, the thymus, and the spleen, refer to one of the newer textbooks such as *Fundamentals of Anatomy and Physiology,* 4 ed.[1] Discussion of the role of lymph nodes in fluid circulation will be expanded in Section III.

Clinical Implications: Patients with negative SLN biopsy results may be spared a complete lymph node dissection. It appears that the SLN biopsy has a lower rate of complications than complete dissections because it is a less invasive procedure. The SLN biopsy, however, does carry some risk. There are reports in the literature and in clinical settings of extremity lymphedema following SLN biopsy.[4] Patients should be educated about lymphedema, risks and precautions, and self-care guidelines regardless of the number of lymph nodes dissected.

FIGURE 1-7 a and b Lymphatic Drainage of the Upper Limb

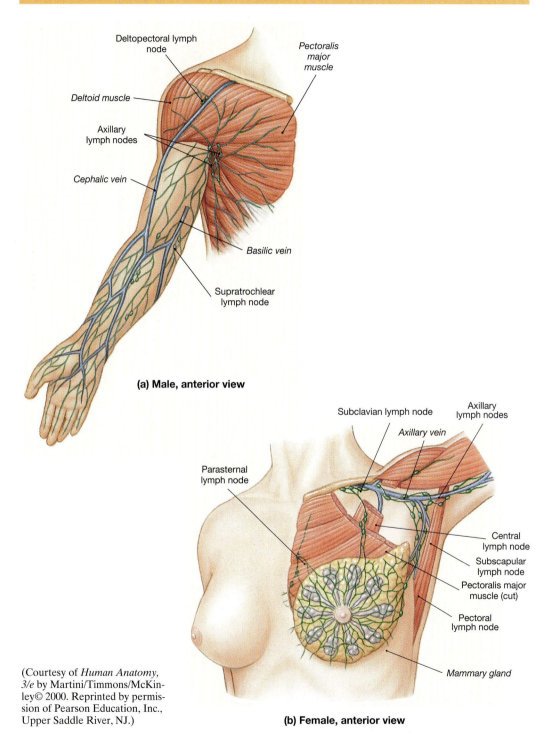

(a) Male, anterior view

(b) Female, anterior view

FIGURE 1-8 Lymphatic Drainage of the Lower Limb

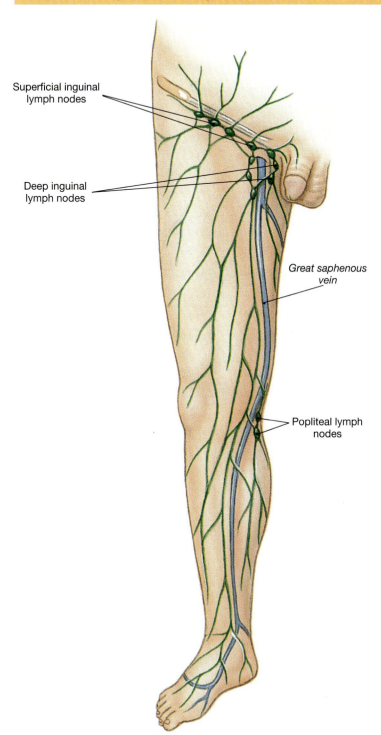

Superficial inguinal lymph nodes

Deep inguinal lymph nodes

Great saphenous vein

Popliteal lymph nodes

(Courtesy of *Human Anatomy, 3/e* by Martini/Timmons/ McKinley© 2000. Reprinted by permission of Pearson Education, Inc., Upper Saddle River, NJ.)

FIGURE 1-9 Lymphatic Drainage of the Inguinal Region

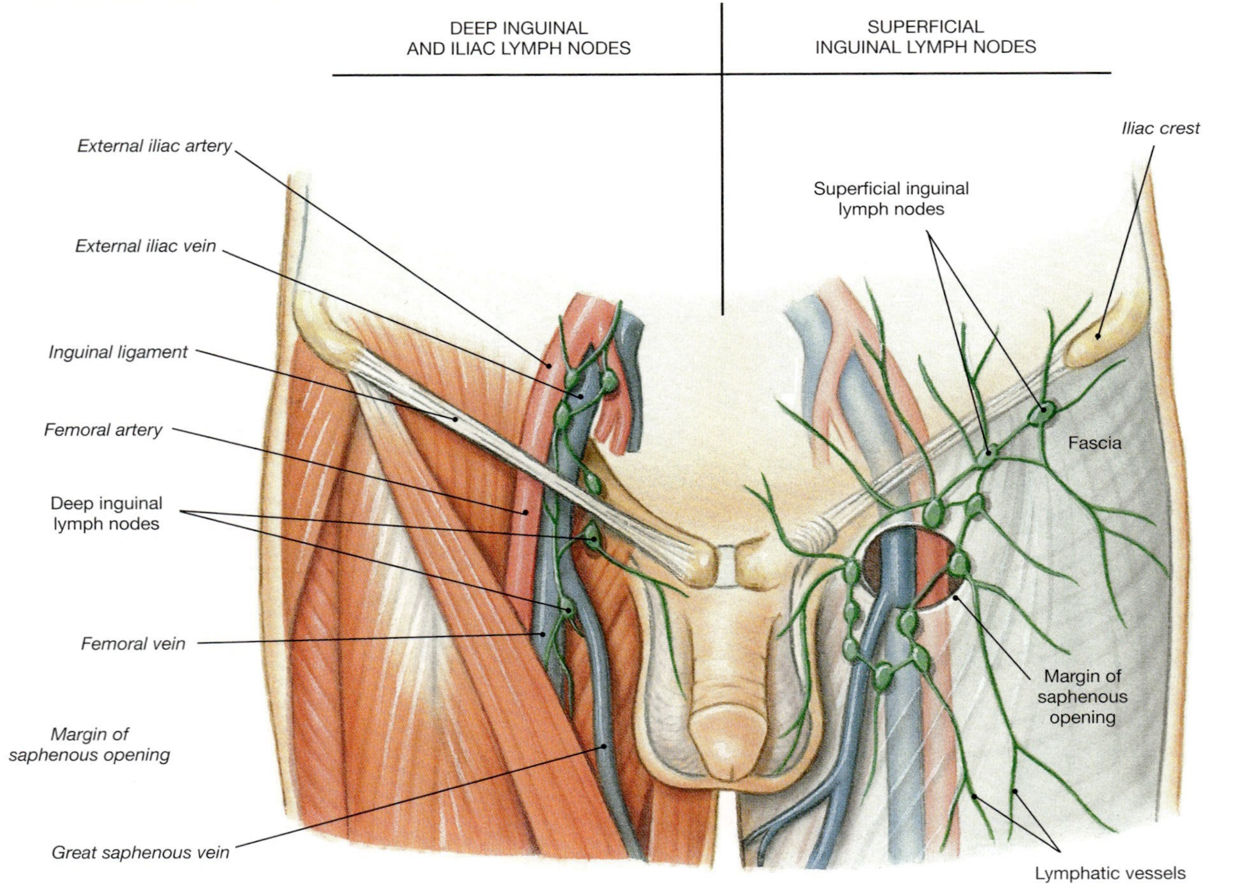

SUPERFICIAL
INGUINAL LYMPH NODES

DEEP INGUINAL
AND ILIAC LYMPH NODES

Iliac crest

Fascia

Margin of
saphenous
opening

Lymphatic vessels

Superficial inguinal
lymph nodes

External iliac artery

External iliac vein

Inguinal ligament

Femoral artery

Deep inguinal
lymph nodes

Femoral vein

Margin of
saphenous opening

Great saphenous vein

Inguinal lymph nodes and vessels

An anterior view of the inguinal lymph nodes and vessels.
(Courtesy of *Human Anatomy, 3/e* by Martini/Timmons/McKinley© 2000. Reprinted by permission of Pearson Education, Inc.. Upper Saddle River, NJ.)

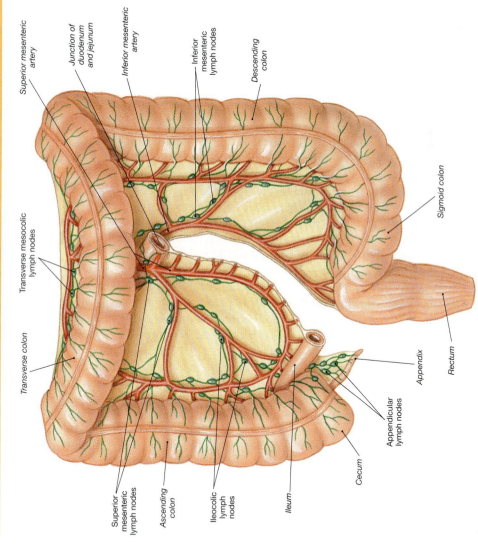

Superior mesenteric artery

Junction of duodenum and jejunum

Inferior mesenteric artery

Inferior mesenteric lymph nodes

Descending colon

Transverse mesocolic lymph nodes

Transverse colon

Sigmoid colon

Rectum

Appendix

Appendicular lymph nodes

Cecum

Ileum

Ileocolic lymph nodes

Ascending colon

Superior mesenteric lymph nodes

(Courtesy of *Human Anatomy, 3/e* by Martini/Timmons/McKinley© 2000. Reprinted by permission of Pearson Education, Inc., Upper Saddle River, NJ.)

D. **Thoracic duct, right lymphatic duct, and lymphovenous anastomoses**
The deep lymphatics merge into larger vessels called *lymphatic trunks.*
The trunks empty into the **thoracic duct** and the **right lymphatic duct**.
The largest lymph vessel in the body is the thoracic duct. The thoracic
duct is crucial in the lymphatic system as it carries three-fourths of the
lymph fluid passing through the body every day. This means that 1 to 2
liters of fluid empty into the left venous angle each day in the normal
individual. The thoracic duct carries lymph from the lower body below
the diaphragm and the left side of the body above the diaphragm. It
originates around the vertebral level of L2 in a "saclike chamber" called
the *cysterna chyli.* The cysterna chyli collects lymph fluid from the lumbar trunks and the intestinal trunk (see Figure 1.11). The thoracic duct
also collects fluid from the left jugular, left subclavian, and left bronchomediastinal *lymphatic trunks* and empties into a junction between the
left subclavian vein and the left jugular vein referred to as the *left venous angle.* Approximately one-fourth of the lymph load is carried from
the right side of the body above the diaphragm, toward the **right lymphatic duct,** and empties into the **right venous angle**. The right lymphatic duct is formed by the right jugular, right subclavian, and right
bronchomediastinal *lymphatic trunks* near the right clavicle. The right
lymphatic duct empties lymph fluid from the right side of the body
above the diaphragm, into a junction between the right subclavian vein
and the right jugular vein called the *right venous angle.*

III. **Lymph circulation**
As recently as 1989, North American researchers were debating whether or
not lymph vessels had the ability to participate in fluid and protein homeostasis. *The investigation and confirmation of how lymph fluid moves from
one place to another has been critical in determining which types of intervention are appropriate when the system fails.* A basic understanding of the various mechanisms of lymph transport will give the clinician an appreciation
of the complexities of the system. A review of pertinent anatomy and physiology will illustrate how superficial and delicate the first level of lymph circulation is. From there, follow the route of lymph fluid as it travels to the
pre-collectors, the deeper collector vessels, through the lymph nodes, and
ultimately to the thoracic duct and left venous angle or the right lymphatic
duct and the right venous angle.
The components of lymph circulation are:
• Microcirculation
• Pre-collectors
• Deep vessels
• Lymph nodes
• Thoracic duct
• Left and right venous angles
A. **Microcirculation**
The two most important fluid exchange processes in microcirculation
are diffusion and filtration/reabsorption:
1.   *Diffusion* is a passive event that occurs when molecules move from
an area of higher concentration to an area of lower concentration,

FIGURE 1-11 Lymphatic Ducts and Lymphatic Drainage

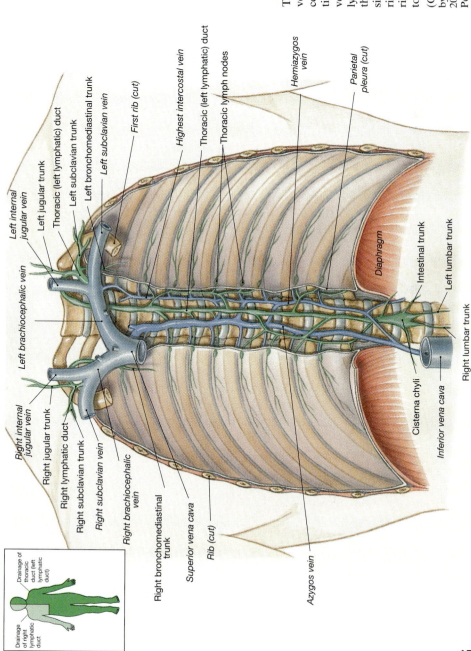

The collecting system of lymph vessels, nodes, major lymphatic collecting ducts and their relationship to the brachiocephalic veins. The thoracic duct collects lymph from tissues inferior to the diaphragm and from the left side of the upper body. The right lymphatic duct drains the right half of the body superior to the diaphragm.

(Courtesy of *Human Anatomy, 3/e* by Martini/Timmons/McKinley© 2000. Reprinted by permission of Pearson Education, Inc., Upper Saddle River, NJ.)

Left internal
jugular vein

Left jugular trunk

Thoracic (left lymphatic) duct

Left subclavian trunk

Left bronchomediastinal trunk

Left subclavian vein

First rib (cut)

Highest intercostal vein

Thoracic (left lymphatic) duct

Thoracic lymph nodes

Hemiazygos vein

Parietal pleura (cut)

Diaphragm

Intestinal trunk

Left lumbar trunk

Right lumbar trunk

Inferior vena cava

Cisterna chyli

Azygos vein

Rib (cut)

Superior vena cava

Right brachiocephalic vein

Right bronchomediastinal trunk

Right subclavian vein

Right subclavian trunk

Right lymphatic duct

Right jugular trunk

Left brachiocephalic vein

Right internal jugular vein

Drainage of thoracic duct (left lymphatic duct)

Drainage of right lymphatic duct

17

thus allowing involved substances to reach equilibrium. Diffusion is important in the constitution of body fluids because it eliminates local concentration gradients. In other words, diffusion keeps body fluids in equilibrium. To be effective, the diffusion rate must keep up with the needs of active cells. There are several factors that influence diffusion rate. Two factors of interest to the clinician are:

a. *Molecule size:* Small molecules diffuse more rapidly than large ones. Protein molecules are large and diffuse more slowly. In the case of a disorder that involves high concentrations of protein molecules, such as lymphedema, compromise to tissue health can arise because of the protein-rich fluid buildup.

b. *Temperature:* The higher the temperature, the faster the diffusion rate. Tissue temperatures can be raised by many influences including infection, inflammation, heavy exercise, heat modalities, and deep-tissue massage.

Clinical Implications: In the impaired lymphatic system, uptake of lymph fluid, including a heavy load of protein molecules, will not be able to keep pace with the demands of the diffusion rate. Every attempt should be made to avoid an increase in tissue temperature because the increase in heat will increase the diffusion rate. Individuals with a lymphatic system at risk should be educated about avoiding exposure to higher temperatures. Interestingly, a few small studies have investigated the use of heat to increase lymphatic vessel function. However, until more is understood about the role heat plays in the health and function of the lymphatic system, clinicians should avoid application of heat modalities to an edematous body region or a limb "at risk." (Refer to Chapter 3 for a description of the limb "at risk.")

In any discussion of diffusion, *osmosis* must be included. This refers to the *net diffusion* of water across a membrane. Since a cell membrane is freely permeable to water, fluid will either flow in or out in order to create an osmotic equilibrium of the solution on both sides of the membrane. Problems will occur if there is an accumulation of protein molecules on one side of a capillary wall. These molecules are too big to pass through the cell membrane, so the water must come to them to create equilibrium. If there is a buildup of protein molecules because the lymphatic system is impaired and cannot remove them fast enough, there will also be a buildup of water molecules as they move toward the higher solute concentration.

The *osmotic pressure* of a solution gives information about the force of water moving into the solution. An opposing pressure is needed to prevent too much osmotic flow of water into a solution. Resisting or pushing against a fluid generates *hydrostatic pressure*. The elastic properties of cutaneous tissues play an important role in resisting osmotic flow or *maintaining tissue hydrostatic pressures*. The loss of skin elasticity through fibrosis, combined with a breakdown in the lymph system fluid transport mechanism, can mean an increase in limb size.

Clinical Implications: Maintaining appropriate levels of hydrostatic pressure can be a therapeutic intervention. In the impaired lymphatic system, application of specific types of external pressure in a careful, controlled fashion can slow *ultrafiltration* (dispersed particles but not the liquid are held back). This could include lymphedema bandaging, the pneumatic pump, and compression garments (see Chapters 4 and 5). An external intervention, such as a compression pump, used without guidance, will cause the removal of water from tissues but will not remove protein molecules. After rapid or forceful removal, water will return to the area and quickly diffuse across the cell membranes in an effort to equilibrate the solutions again, thus increasing the edema.

Understanding hydrostatic pressure can also be important for prevention and control guidelines for the person who has lymphedema or is at risk of developing lymphedema. Due to the positive effects of gentle pressure, the hydrostatic pressure of water makes swimming an excellent exercise for the person "at risk" or the person who has lymphedema. Principles of hydrostatic pressure may also explain why air travel has been identified as a factor in precipitating or exacerbating the symptoms of lymphedema in some individuals. The decrease in pressure inside the airplane cabin allows an increase in ultrafiltration in the body. To an already impaired system, combined with other factors involving air travel such as immobility, this may be the final insult that puts a portion of the lymphatic system into permanent failure.

2. *Filtration* and *reabsorption* are closely linked with diffusion, osmosis, and hydrostatic pressure. *Filtration* occurs when hydrostatic pressure forces water across a membrane. Water is pushed from an area of high pressure to an area of lower pressure. Solute molecules may cross with the water if they are small enough. Large molecules, like protein, will stay behind because they cannot cross the membrane via filtration. Blood pressure is actually the hydrostatic pressure of the blood and is often referred to as blood hydrostatic pressure (BHP), or in the capillaries as blood capillary pressure (BCP). Along the length of a typical capillary, blood pressure gradually falls and is the lowest at the start of the venous system. *Filtration* occurs primarily at the arterial end where the BHP is highest.

    Reabsorption occurs as a result of osmosis, which was discussed in the preceding paragraph. The osmotic pressure is referred to as (OP), or (COP) for colloid osmotic pressure, or (BCOP) for blood colloid osmotic pressure. The term *oncotic pressure* is also used for BCOP and is equally acceptable. Remember that the osmotic pressure of a solution refers to the force of water molecule movement toward the solution containing a higher solute concentration.

Following the interactions between filtration and reabsorption along a capillary, you will begin to see how some clinical interventions will assist the lymphatic system and some could work against it. *Reminder:* Hydrostatic pressure forces water *out* of a solution, while osmotic pressure draws water *into* a solution. In the normal system, there is a fine balance between outward pressure or BHP and inward pressure or BCOP on the capillary system. This balance was identified by E.H. Starling and is called *Starling's Law* (or *Starling's Equilibrium)*. In simple terms, you can remember this law as "more in = more out."[1] *There is continual movement of fluid from the bloodstream into the tissues and back to the bloodstream via the lymphatic system.* The rates of filtration and reabsorption slowly change as blood passes along the length of a capillary. BHP tends to be higher at the arterial end of a capillary, while BCOP tends to be lower toward the venous end of the capillary. This allows water and solutes to be pulled into the venous system. Approximately 24 liters of fluid moves out of the plasma and into the interstitial fluid every 24 hours. Of that, 85 to 90% is reabsorbed. The remaining 10 to 15%, or 2 to 4 liters, flows through the tissues and into lymphatic vessels for eventual return to the venous system.[1,5]

If BHP rises or BCOP falls (more out=less in), fluid will move out of the blood and into the nearby tissues resulting in edema. If the lymphatic system becomes permanently overloaded and unable to remove excess fluid adequately, the final consequence will be lymphedema.

Many individuals who present with damage to the lymphatic system will not develop lymphedema. Due to a large functional reserve, the lymphatic system can work much harder than it does under normal conditions. This functional reserve allows most individuals to recover from episodes of excess fluid in the interstitium without permanent changes in lymphatic function.

Clinicians who are certified (receive specific education) in lymphedema management are well versed in the specialized functions of the lymph system including *transport capacity, lymph load, lymph time volume,* and *safety valve function.* For a more in-depth explanation of these functions, seek out a medical professional with specialized education in lymphedema management, or a physician specializing in lymphology or vascular pathologies. (See Chapter 8 for contacts.)

Clinical Implications: Will your intervention improve or assist the balance between BHP and BCOP? Be cautious about the use of high, external pressures such as the compression pump or garment, vigorous massage, string wrapping, or long-stretch elastic wrapping, which may temporarily, mechanically remove water from the tissues of a limb, leaving protein molecules behind only to attract more water. Deep-tissue treatments may also cause focal damage to the lymphatics—primarily the endothelial lining.[6] Since capillary dynamics begin immediately below the surface of the skin, which of your interventions might be occluding capillary flow or causing cell death or obstruction? As you will read in Chapter 4, there are treatments that can work in harmony with cell physiology and support the function of deeper lymphatic structures. Variations in total tissue pressure assist with the function of the superficial and deep lymphatic vessels. Specialized manual techniques can assist by providing variations in tissue pressure.

B. **Precollectors** contribute to lymph circulation by channeling fluids that have been absorbed toward the vessels that will transport them into the thoracic duct and right lymphatic duct. Precollectors can move fluid by

FIGURE 1-12 Forces Acting across Capillary Walls

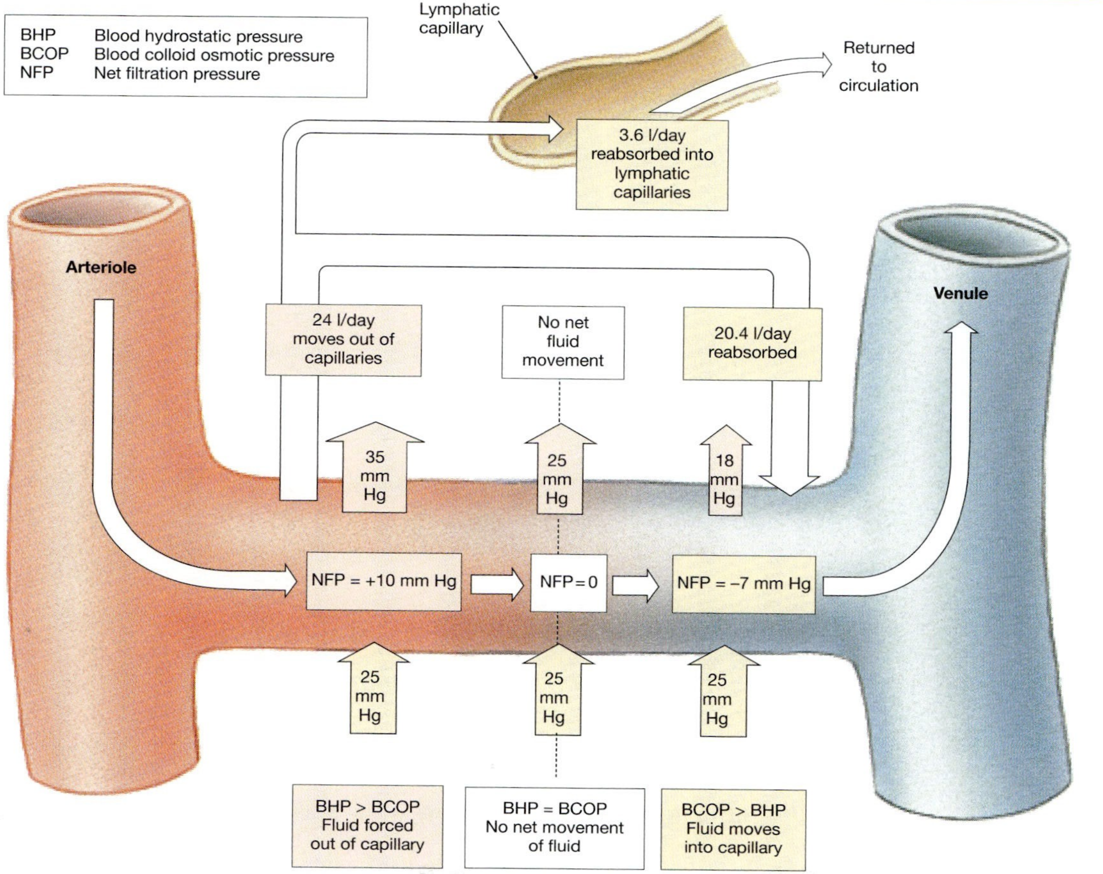

At the arterial end of the capillary, blood hydrostatic pressure (BHP) is stronger than blood colloid osmotic pressure (BCOP), and fluid moves out of the capillary. Near the venule, BHP is lower than BCOP, and fluid moves into the capillary. In this model, interstitial fluid osmotic pressure (ICOP) and interstitial fluid hydrostatic pressure (IHP) are assumed to be 0 mm Hg.

(Courtesy of Fundamentals of Anatomy and Physiology, 4/e by Martini© 1998. Reprinted by permission of Pearson Education, Inc., Upper Saddle River, NJ 07458.)

absorption like capillaries, and through contraction of valves like deeper vessels.

C. **Deep vessels** are divided into segments by valves. The segments between the valves are called *lymphangions*. Lymphangions transport lymph via intrinsic contractions. The heart does not produce a driving force for the lymph. The force is generated by the lymphangions, which act like tiny hearts or lymph pumps.[7] Vessels contract 6 to 10 times per minute at rest but can increase to 10 times faster during exercise.[5] Lymphangions are stimulated to contract segmentally, and thus empty, via a variety of mechanisms:

- Nervous system stimulation. Sympathetic, parasympathetic, and sensory nerve endings are located in the lymph vessels and lymph nodes. These can regulate contractile function.[8] Pain and stress, for example, can influence the activity of the vessels and nodes.
- Contractions of adjacent muscles
- Pulsation of adjacent arteries
- Changes in abdominal and thoracic pressure during breathing
- Lower blood capillary pressure in deep veins
- Lymph vessel volume: Emptying is facilitated after a lymphangion has reached its maximum volume. Internal receptors signal the start of a contraction due to tension on the inner wall of each segment, pushing the fluid into the next segment.
- Mechanical stimulation or traction:[9] External pressures used in the techniques of manual lymph drainage would be an example of mechanical stimulation and are discussed in Chapter 4.

Under certain conditions, lymph is able to flow backward from deep to superficial. This can be seen when transport is impeded in the deeper vessels. It is sometimes referred to as *dermal backflow*. The initial lymphatics become flooded and microlymphatic hypertension increases.[10]

D. **Lymph nodes:** Deeper vessels deliver lymph into the lymph nodes from *afferent* (inflowing) lymph vessels. Lymph is filtered before it leaves the node via *efferent* (outflowing) lymph vessels, heading toward the venous system. In addition to filtering, lymph nodes also play a part in the regulation of protein concentration in lymph fluid. The nodes contribute to the control of hydrostatic pressure, which can cause the addition or subtraction of water as needed to maintain equilibrium in the surrounding tissues.

Clinical Implications: Every lymph node receives, monitors, and filters lymph fluid originating from specific regions of the body. In some individuals, the loss of even one node can trigger the onset of lymphedema in the nearby region. Others are able to accommodate for the loss of many nodes and not suffer permanent signs and symptoms. It is possible for fluid to circumvent an existing lymph node but it is very difficult for it to pass through a region where a lymph node has been dissected and scar tissue has formed. Rerouting the direction of lymph flow utilizing anastomoses and collateral vessels can be achieved with specialized manual techniques, which will be discussed in Chapter 4.

FIGURE 1-13 Drainage Possibilities of the Lymph from a Congested Territory, Moving across the Watershed, to a Normal Territory

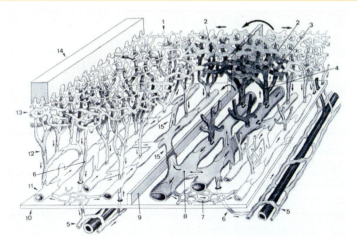

1 Normal capillary network **2** Dilated capillary network **3** Dilated lymph capillaries and pre-collectors **4** Pre-collector which transports fluid backward (dermal backflow-collector to pre-collector-to capillary) **5** Deep lymph collectors **6** Collector perforating muscle and fascia **7** Dilated network of lymph vessels due to congestion **8** Dilated lymph collector **9** Watershed **10** Fascia **11** Normal collector **12** Normal pre-collector **13** Corium network **14** Epidermis **14** Anastomosis connection between superficial collectors

Földi M, Kubik S, *Lehrbuch der Lymphologie*, Gustav Fischer Verlag, 1999. (Courtesy of Urban & Fischer Verlag, Copyright by Urban & Fischer Verlag)

E. **Thoracic duct:** The thoracic duct penetrates the diaphragm on its way from the cysterna chyli to the venous angles. Fluid movement is facilitated through the thoracic duct via most of the same supporting mechanisms as the deep vessels. Pressure changes in the thoracoabdominal region will play a larger role in fluid movement here than elsewhere. A drop in intrathoracic pressure occurs with abdominal breathing and creates a suction force that can facilitate lymphatic flow.[11]
    Clinical Implications: Because deep breathing will facilitate movement of fluid along the thoracic duct, it should be a part of every intervention for edema and lymphedema. Specialized manual techniques can further increase vessel contractions and enhance evacuation of abdominal and pelvic congestion.

F. **Left and right venous angles:** The junctions of the left and right venous angles are distinguished as locations where venous pressure is low enough to allow lymph fluid to flow into the venous system. The normal venous system will handle the additional fluid volume with much of the excess leaving the body in urine.
    Clinical Implications: An individual receiving effective treatment for swelling may report the need to urinate more frequently than usual. The patient may need to interrupt a treatment session to use the restroom or may report that nighttime trips to the bathroom have increased. This is a temporary situation while the body adjusts to the increase in circulating fluid volumes.

The majority of lymph fluid enters the venous system as outlined here: from superficial capillary absorption to precollector, to large vessel contraction, eventually emptying into the venous system. There are, however, lymphovenous anastomoses or connections between the collecting lymphatics and the blood circulating system, which occur in many places, allowing small amounts of lymph to enter the bloodstream in less obvious locations.[2,12]

The diverse means used for moving lymph fluid between cells, from smaller to larger vessels, and through deep vessels to the thoracic duct, attest to the importance of the lymphatic system and its role in transporting fluid loads and managing fluid overloads. Because of the large volume of fluid that is moved by the lymphatic system each day, it is easy to see that a disruption in the system will have a dramatic effect on the health and construction of the tissues in the area.

IV. Connective Tissue Fibrosis

The function of the normal lymphatic system and its multiple methods of moving lymph fluid have been reviewed. Discussion has included several ways in which the system may fail and fluid accumulation may be triggered. The next step is to look at the tissue response to this accumulation of fluid.

A. **Pathophysiology:** In the course of lymphedema development, the concentrated proteins in the interstitial fluid act as foreign bodies, stimulating chronic inflammation and proliferation of connective tissue. Chronic

---

FIGURE 1-14 The Skin

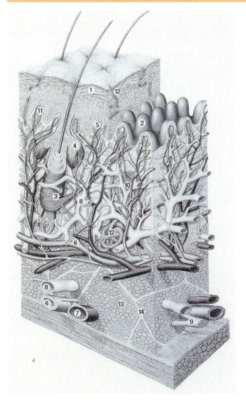

(From Asmussen PD, Sölner B. *Wound Healing* Published by Hippokrates, Stuttgart, 1993) **1** Stratum corneum (epidermis) **2** Papillae **3** Hair follicle **4** Sebaceous gland **5** Capillary loop of the initial lymphatics **6** Pre-capillary arteriole **7** Post-capillary venule **8** Lymph collector **9** Nerve **10** Pacinian corpuscle **11** Meissner's corpuscle **12** Sweat gland with duct **13** Subcutaneous adipose tissue **14** Collagen fiber
Földi M, Kubik S, *Lehrbuch der Lymphologie*, Gustav Fischer Verlag, 1999.

(Courtesy of Urban & Fischer Verlag, Copyright by Urban & Fischer Verlag)

inflammation plus the metabolic disturbance resulting from lymph flow failure cause tissues to react, forming a network of fibrosclerotic tissue.[13] The balance between the deposition and lysis of collagenous fibers is shifted in favor of deposition. Initially, deposition of fibrosclerotic tissue is in the area surrounding the affected lymphatic vessels. As fibrous tissue builds, endothelial cells become functionally impaired. The fibrosclerotic tissue is an impedance to diffusion, osmosis, and consequently, the control of hydrostatic pressure. More protein accumulates, more fibrous tissue is formed, often in the vessel walls, as the condition extends out from the affected vessels. *At this point, many individuals still do not exhibit clinical signs and symptoms, yet the system is now seriously impaired.*

The continual progression of fibrosclerotic tissue causes a reduction in the transport capacity of the entire remaining system. At any time along this continuum, a sudden increase in the amount of lymph waiting to be transported may trigger a permanent failure in the system in some individuals. The sudden increase in lymph could occur due to a variety of triggers including examples such as vigorous exercise, a skin wound, air travel, or a local infection. (See Chapters 2 through 4 for additional discussion and references.) *Lymphedema would now be clinically evident and measurable.* Left untreated, proteins and cellular debris continue to accumulate, fibrosclerotic tissue continues to accumulate, and a cycle of inflammation, infection, and limb enlargement will begin.

B. **Other inflammatory mediators:** Protein-rich stagnant lymph fluid is blamed as the primary inflammatory mediator in infection and the frequent bouts of infection such as cellulitis, which patients with lymphedema often suffer. Protein molecules precipitate potent oncotic pressures but are not the only culprits. Fatty acids have oncotic pressure. Leukocytes spew out their waste and create an inflamed environment as well. There is much investigation yet to be done to enhance our understanding of the inflammatory process and its impact on the lymphatic system.

C. **Radiation therapy:** Radiation can independently damage the lymphatics and blood vessels, as well as skin and subcutaneous tissues.[14] Radiation induced injury to the vascular system may also contribute to some of the chronic fibrotic changes associated with lymphedema.[15]

D. **Other types of edema:** Any type of edema can lead to tissue fibrosis and infection, causing symptoms similar to lymphedema including: pain, feelings of pressure, disfigurement, and functional disability. Edema fluid reduces oxygenation of tissues, impairs cellular function, and delays healing. This in turn reduces mobility and creates risk of injury and infection. *Edema fluid with high levels of protein, however, injures tissues more than fluid with low levels of protein.*

Clinical Implications: The progression of lymphedema from the first signs and symptoms to irreversible fibrotic changes takes time. It is easier to effect changes in this process earlier rather than later. Early accurate diagnosis, patient education, and appropriate treatment will decrease the amount of time needed to achieve limb reduction, skin

Natural progression of an impaired lymph system: lymph stasis	
Morphological Changes	*Patient Response*
Insult to lymph vessels or nodes.	**Acute edema** may last 4–6 weeks.
Rapid bridging of the gap by **new lymphatics,** lymph drainage restored.[16] **Alternative drainage pathways** are established. Variations in vessels among individuals will assure that some will have **collateral circulation** to rely on after the removal of axillary or inguinal lymph nodes while others will not.[5]	**No edema** Evidence exists that shows that some individuals will respond with compensation and the formation of new vessels and pathways, which can prevent the onset of lymphedema.[17]
In the absence of adequate lymph drainage for any reason there will be **growing lymph stasis**	**No edema, or may develop** at any time if the morphological processes occur rapidly. Can occur within months or years of insult.
Progressive structural changes in soft tissue. Fibrosis of lymphatics and surrounding connective tissue, loss of vessel permeability, dilatation of lymph vessels, valvular incompetencies, incompetent interendothelial junctions (flaps) in lymph capillaries, skin laxity, decreased effectiveness of muscle pump, exhaustion of macrophage activity, **continued growing lymph stasis.**	Up to 30% fluid overload may occur before swelling is visible. **Patient may complain** of feeling of heaviness, pain, tingling, or numbness **or may appear clinically normal with no complaints.** In two studies, patients who remained asymptomatic at two or more years post insult had radiographic signs of decompensation in their involved limb.[15,16]
Permanent, chronic fluid overload of the impaired lymph system. Infiltration of fibroblasts, deposition of collagen continues.	**Visible swelling,** decline in skin integrity, rise in rate of infection in involved limb, increase in patient complaints of feeling of heaviness, loss of motion, pain, tingling, numbness, cosmetic issues, decrease in quality of life.
In the absence of accurate diagnosis and/or adequate treatment, progressive tissue changes continue.	If no treatment is administered, the **patient is at risk** of repeated infections, cellulitis, increased swelling, loss of mobility, and risk of malignancy, eventually reaching Stage 3 or *elephantiasis.* Symptom progression rate varies per individual. **Note the importance of early diagnosis, patient education, and appropriate treatment.**
Elephantiasis following prolonged destruction of lymph vessels and obliteration of lymph nodes. Usually but not always seen following repeated attacks of secondary acute inflammation/infection.	Skin has a grotesque appearance, hard to the touch, and discolored. Involved limb can be more than double the size of the uninvolved side. Papillomas are common. Patient suffers profound loss of function.

changes, and overall improvement in function. *Due to the importance of early intervention to the long-term management of the signs and symptoms, patients should not be allowed to languish in settings that cannot appropriately diagnose and treat lymphedema.* Referring practitioners and their patients should be directed toward locations where lymphedema is routinely treated with current intervention methods. See Chapter 8 for information on how to find these locations.

References

1. Martini, F. H. 1989. *Fundamentals of Anatomy and Physiology,* 4th ed. Upper Saddle River, NJ: Prentice Hall.
2. Casley-Smith, J. R. 1980. The fine structure and functioning of tissue channels and lymphatics. *Lymphology* 12:177–83.
3. Szuba, A. and Rockson, S. G. 1997. Lymphedema: Anatomy, physiology and pathogenesis. *Vasc Med.* 2:321–26.
4. Wrone, D. A. et al. 2000. Lymphedema after sentinel lymph node biopsy for cutaneous melanoma. *Arch Dermatol.* 136:511–14.
5. Weissleder, H. and Schuchhardt, C. 1997. *Lymphedema Diagnosis and Therapy,* 2nd ed. Bonn, Germany: Kagerer Kommunication.
6. Eliska, O. and Eliskova, M. 1995. Are peripheral lymphatics damaged by high pressure manual massage? *Lymphology* 28:21–30.
7. Földi, M. 1998. Are there enigmas concerning the pathophysiology of lymphedema after breast cancer treatment? *NLN Newsletter* 10(4):1–4.
8. Hukkanen, M., Konttinen, Y. T., Terenghi, G., Polak, J. M. 1992. Peptide-containing innervation of rat femoral lymphatic vessels. *Microvasc Res.* 43(1):7–19.
9. Tunkel, R. and Cohen, S. 2000. Lymphedema management. *Rehabilitation Oncology* 18(1): 26–27.
10. Franzeck, et al. 1997. Combined physical therapy for lymphedema evaluated by fluorescence microlymphography and lymph capillary pressure measurements. *J Vasc Res.* 34:306–11.
11. Wittlinger, H. 1989. *Textbook of Dr. Vodder's Manual Lymphatic Drainage II.* Heidelberg, Germany: Karl R. Hang Publishers.
12. Földi, M. 1977. The lymphatic system. A review. *J Lymphology* (1)16–19, 44–56.
13. Piller, N. B. 1980. Lymphoedema, macrophages and benzopyrones. *Lymphology* 13:109–19.
14. Tsyb, A. F., Bardychev, M. S., Guseva, L. I. 1981. Secondary limb edema following irradiation. *Lymphology* 14:127–32.
15. Brennan, M. F. 1992. Lymphedema following the surgical treatment of breast cancer: A review of pathophysiology and treatment. *J Pain Symptom Manage.* 7:110–16.
16. Olszewski, W. 1973. On the pathomechanism of development of postsurgical lymphedema. *Lymphology* 6:35–51.
17. Goltner, E., Gass, P., Hass, J. P., Schneider, P. 1988. The importance of volumetry, lymphscintigraphy and computer tomography in the diagnosis of brachial edema after mastectomy. *Lymphology* 21:134–43.

2
LYMPHEDEMA

"In the past, physicians always played down the importance of lymphedema and pointed out to generations of patients that it is very rare, that there is no effective treatment, that the patient must learn to 'live with it,' or even that it will get better some day or will go away. Moreover, physicians have failed to instruct patients on how to avoid lymphedema after surgery or radiation therapy, and continue to grossly understate the incidence of this very serious and life-long illness."

DR. ROBERT LERNER

INTRODUCTION

Now that normal lymphatic system function has been briefly outlined, it is easier to understand what happens when the system is unable to function normally. Lymphedema is a chronic disorder that is characterized by an abnormal accumulation of lymph fluid in the tissues of an extremity or other body part. The accumulation of fluid is most often due to a mechanical insufficiency of the lymphatic system. In other words, the available lymphatic components are not functioning sufficiently to manage the load of lymph fluid that is present in the system. There are many potential causes for the insufficiency including but not limited to problems with:

- vessel walls (hyperplasia, hypoplasia)
- valves (unable to close)
- collector vessel obstruction (scar tissue, tumor)
- lymphangion contraction (spasm or paralysis)
- node or vessel absence (congenital or secondary to dissection)
- node or vessel disruption or damage (radiation, surgery, or trauma)
- disease processes that involve veins or lymphatics (chronic venous insufficiency, rheumatoid arthritis)

For a more in-depth look at the pathogenesis of lymphedema, refer to works by Földi,[1] Szuba,[2] Casley-Smith,[3] and Brennan.[4]

Potential anatomical locations of lymphedema include all areas where lymph nodes and vessels are located: the extremities, head and neck, chest, back, genitalia, and abdomen. The spinal cord and brain are not directly supplied with lymph nodes or vessels, so are not affected. The signs and symptoms of lymphedema may include any or all of the following:

- swelling
- great discomfort (often described as pain)
- numbness and/or tingling

- sensation of pressure or tightness of skin or limb
- heaviness of limb
- increased susceptibility to infection
- fibrotic changes to the skin and underlying connective tissues
- lymphatic cysts or fistulas, lymphorrhea, papillomas, hyperkeratinosis
- loss of mobility
- impaired wound healing

Any combination of these signs or symptoms may have an impact on the individual's quality of life and functional ability.

Although a permanent condition, when treated appropriately, the signs and symptoms can be reduced and managed. In many cases, when early intervention is combined with a patient who adheres to the recommended program, symptoms appear to be reversed. If managed inappropriately, signs and symptoms may remain the same but most often progress to a more serious stage.[5] If untreated, tissue fibrosis and system decline is progressive. Untreated lymphedema may result in lymphangiosar-coma.[1,2] This malignant tumor, also known as *Stewart-Treves Syndrome,* can arise as a complication of lymphedema. Kaposi's sarcoma may also result from long-standing lymphedema.[6]

ETIOLOGY

The *etiology* or *initial cause* of the condition should not be confused with the *initiating factor* or *stimulus*, which starts the actual lymphedema for each individual. Both will be discussed in this chapter. The etiology of lymphedema is currently divided or classified into two major categories: *primary* and *secondary lymphedema.*

Primary lymphedema is thought to be caused by a condition that is either congenital or hereditary. Complications to the developing fetus can be a factor as well. There are such variations from person to person that some investigators are reluctant to state that primary lymphedema is completely understood. In primary lymphedema, lymph vessel or lymph node development has been impaired. Although a variety of dysplasias may present themselves, *hypoplasia* is the most common cause of problems. With hypoplasia, there are fewer lymphatics present and they are smaller than normal. Two of the more common types of primary lymphedema have been identified as *Milroy's Disease* and *Meige's Syndrome.* Refer to the literature for a more extensive look at these and other conditions associated with primary lymphedema.[2,7,8] (See Figures 2.2, 2.5, and 2.6.)

Other key points about primary lymphedema of interest to the clinician include:

- 83% manifest before age 35 and are called lymphedema praecox[5]
- 17% manifest after age 35 and are called lymphedema tardum
- 87% of all cases of primary lymphedema occur in females[5]
- Onset occurs most often around age 17 or during puberty (but can be present at birth)
- Lower extremities are more often involved than other body parts

Once the signs and symptoms appear, primary lymphedema, like secondary, usually develops progressively without adequate intervention and management.

Symptoms are triggered or exacerbated by events such as heat, pregnancy, trauma, and local infections. Initiating factors for all types of lymphedema will be examined further after the discussion of secondary lymphedema.

Secondary lymphedema is caused by the result of some known insult to the lymphatic system. Lymph capillaries, vessels, and/or nodes have been removed, blocked, fibrosed, damaged, or necrosed and have become insufficient to manage the lymph load that has accumulated in the involved body part. Worldwide, secondary lymphedema is more common than primary. The most common causes of secondary lymphedema include:

- **Surgery:** Cancer-related surgeries of the breast, prostate, bladder, uterus, or skin usually dissect or disrupt lymph nodes and vessels. Most studies have established a correlation between the degree of axillary dissection and the likelihood of developing lymphedema. There is an abundance of literature indicating a correlation between inguinal dissection and lower extremity lymphedema as well.[9–17] Surgical dissection of lymph nodes and vessels will challenge the remaining lymphatics. In some individuals, the collateral vessels are inadequate to manage lymph circulation and lymphedema will result. In some cases, even patients undergoing limited axillary dissection, as in a lumpectomy, develop lymphedema. (See Figure 2.3.)
- **Radiation therapy** contributes to fibrosis of involved tissues, which leads to a decrease in circulation of lymph fluid in the involved area. Radiation also decreases the availability of collateral pathways for fluid removal. Radiation shrinks lymph nodes and can render those nodes unable to respond to trauma or infection. X-rays also hinder the regeneration of lymph vessels.[18] These changes will have an impact on the likelihood that a person will develop lymphedema following radiation therapy.[19–23]
- **Trauma** to a region of the body with lymph nodes or key vessels may lead to lymphedema. Pelvic fracture, liposuction, brachial plexus injury, or thermal injury may involve components of the lymphatic system. Trauma can reduce the transport capacity of the lymphatics to below the level of the normal lymphatic fluid load, causing the signs of early lymphedema.[18]
- **Filariasis** is endemic in tropical and subtropical regions of the world. Nematode worm larvae are transmitted to humans by mosquito bites. Adult filaria live, reproduce, and die in the lymphatic vessels. It is currently thought that the death of the parasite causes local inflammation, followed by chronic inflammation, damaged, and blocked lymph vessels.[8] (See Figure 2.4.)
- **Benign or malignant tumor growth** may block circulation of a lymph node or vessel. Malignant tumors may also metastasize to lymph nodes, blocking flow of lymph fluid.
- **Iatrogenic alterations** damage lymph nodes or vessels by diagnostic or therapeutic measures. Examples are hernia repair, by-pass surgery, dissection of any region with lymph nodes or key vessels, such as the knee, neck, or abdomen.[5]
- **Infection** that occurs for any reason worsens edema by increasing local blood flow and capillary permeability, sending more fluid to an overloaded and impaired lymphatic system. In addition, localized infections will

contribute to tissue destruction and increased fibrosis, potentially leading to lymphedema.[4,24]

- **Chronic venous insufficiency** can aggravate or initiate symptoms of lymphedema due to fluid overload from diseased veins.[25,26]
- **Self-induced or artificial lymphedema** has been identified in European literature[8] in which individuals artificially cause the lymphedema. Lymph flow is most often obstructed with a tourniquet to produce signs and symptoms.

UNDERSTANDING THE "LIMB AT RISK"

Millions of people around the world sustain disruption of the lymphatic system and each of them is at risk of developing lymphedema. Many will never experience the onset of the condition. While knowledge of the predictors of onset continues to grow, the ability to accurately predict who will develop the symptoms does not yet exist. Precautions must be observed, therefore, by everyone who is at risk in order to prevent as many cases as possible. *Due to the unique variations in lymphatic anatomy for each individual, the damage and subsequent tissue changes that lead to signs and symptoms may take months or years to appear clinically*. Those who have already developed lymphedema should use the same list of precautions to control or avoid exacerbations of their symptoms as those who are "at risk."

The parts of the body at risk for developing lymphedema will most often be those surrounding and distal to lymph vessel disruption. The body parts most often affected by lymphedema are the extremities due to disruption of axillary or inguinal lymph nodes and/or vessels. The term *limb at risk* serves as a reference for the extremity closest to the lymph vessel disruption. Any part of the body supplied by the lymphatic system and subsequently disrupted can be at risk. When a person is given a list of precautions or guidelines for the care of an extremity, the same instructions can be applied to any other body part at risk such as the head, neck, trunk, abdomen, or genital regions. For example, a person who has had surgery and radiation for prostate cancer will apply the precautions to his abdominal, genital, and lower extremity regions. A person who has had treatment for cancer of the throat would apply the precautions to the head, neck, and trunk.

RISK FOR LYMPHEDEMA: PREDISPOSING FACTORS

Lymphedema should not be considered an inevitable side effect of cancer treatment, trauma, or venous insufficiency. Some individuals have adequate, existing collateral circulation to manage the extra lymph load even with a mechanically insufficient system. For some, lymph vessel regeneration occurs, assuring sufficient lymph circulation. For others, it is an avoidable condition given early, thorough patient education on prevention and control. At this time, health professionals are not able to predict with certainty who will develop the condition. Every person at risk should receive adequate education and the tools to attempt to prevent or control the symptoms.

In the literature there is a common list of prevention and control guidelines that has been circulating for many years. The National Lymphedema Network (NLN) has a list titled "18 Steps to Prevention" that can be accessed on their website; Chapter 8 also includes a list of prevention and control guidelines that readers may copy and distribute to patients. The prevention and control measures are sensible suggestions that do not require drastic life changes and could apply to most individuals wanting to practice a healthy lifestyle. Many of these factors focus around protection of the skin to prevent infection, a common cause of the onset of lymphedema. The list has been created over time and is based on clinical observation, patient reports, and anecdotal,[a] empirical,[b] and scientific[c] information.

Currently, investigators are looking at the most common risk factors and prevention and control guidelines with the intent of collecting evidence-based information.[27] Of concern at this point is the issue that patients at risk may be told by some practitioners to resume a normal lifestyle because evidence supporting the prevention and control guidelines has not been collected using scientific methodology. Many lymphedema management experts agree with Dr. Michael Földi that ". . . there are cases in which 'anecdotal observations' are in harmony with scientific fact and established knowledge."[18] For example, one of the commonly practiced precautions is to avoid sunburn and sunbathing. Many patients have reported excessive exposure led to the onset of lymphedema. Földi states, "It is textbook knowledge that healthy elastic fibers are pre-requisite for lymph formation and that sunshine can destroy those elastic fibers, leading to lymphedema. To try to achieve an evidence-based study would be unethical."[18] There is a need for additional collection of data. Some of the studies examining current predictors or risk factors have collected information on only a single patient population: those treated for breast cancer.[28] Additionally, many patients have co-morbidities, which contribute to or aggravate the signs and symptoms of lymphedema, especially when combined with an event such as surgery or radiation for cancer. Diagnoses such as rheumatoid arthritis, chronic venous insufficiency, hypertension, and lipedema may be predisposing factors not previously addressed in the prevention and control guidelines.

During this period of ongoing investigation, patients must be informed about the risk factors and preventative measures as they are currently understood, and assisted in how to interpret current available information. To educate patients on how to assess the prevention and control guidelines, clinicians should advise patients to *avoid activities that can trigger a further decrease of the transport capacity of the lymph vessels and/or unnecessarily increase the lymphatic fluid and protein load of the lymphatic system in the affected region.*[18] Patients without a medical background may need assistance in understanding what this means in practical and applicable terms. A good place to start is with the current guidelines, which follow the precautions described above. The treatment intervention described in Chapter 4 is also compatible with this advice.

For a person who has had disruption to the lymphatic system via one of the events listed previously under *secondary lymphedema,* the following risk factors may make it more likely that lymphedema will develop at some point:

---

[a]based on experience
[b]based on individual cases
[c]based on measurement and analysis of verifiable data

Age:

For at least a decade data has seemed to imply that the older a person is when the lymphatic system insult occurs, the more likely they are to develop lymphedema. This is explained by the slowing of all circulation systems, and the less efficient uptake of all fluids due to aging. While this may still be true, new trends are not as clear cut. In two studies in the last 10 years with patients following breast cancer, age did not appear to play a significant role in development of lymphedema.[7,29] Other studies identify age as likely to influence progression of lymphedema after its onset.[30] Aging decreases the force of the lymph pumps. Fatigue and structural changes in the vessels will result. Remaining lymphatics take on the work load of the missing or weakened lymph pumps and may be unable to efficiently manage this increased load.[18]

Obesity:

The connection between the onset of lymphedema and obesity relates to the assumption that there are connections between blood, lymph circulation, and the formation of adipose tissue. Slower circulation will lead to the biosynthesis of fat, while faster circulation will lead to lipolysis.[31] In a study at Memorial Sloan-Kettering Breast Service, Dr. Jeanne A. Petrek states, "We already knew that infection and obesity contribute to the onset of lymphedema, but we were surprised to learn that weight gain following a cancer diagnosis is an especially high risk factor."[32] Patients should be advised to achieve or maintain normal weight to avoid this risk factor. Further information on the new relationship between obesity and lymphedema should be available in the scientific literature in the next few years.

Infection:

Onset or exacerbation of lymphedema may be provoked by a local inflammatory response that may occur with infection. Skin flora invade the system through a portal of entry caused by a variety of seemingly minor incidents. The already present, protein-rich fluid facilitates bacterial growth. In the impaired system, this may trigger a fluid and waste component overload that the system cannot remove on its own. For those who do not develop lymphedema after an infection, the cumulative effects of repeated infections can bring a person closer to the threshold of lymphatic system tolerance with each episode.[13,33]

INITIATING FACTORS

In review, a regional lymphatic network that has been subjected to insult has had its capacity to transport and filter the lymphatic load diminished. This reduced capacity may not be enough to result immediately in the swelling characteristic of lymphedema. From that point on, however, lymph stasis may be present. Any activity or event that directly or indirectly further impairs the transport capacity or increases the lymph load has the potential to trigger the onset of lymphedema—at first mild, but leading to swelling that is visible, palpable, measurable, and chronic.

The *stimulus* or *trigger* that causes the initial onset of the symptoms of lymphedema will be different for each person. From the evidence and information that has been collected, there are some trends worth noting. Triggers have been placed in common categories with selected examples to illustrate the possibilities. Information has been gleaned from the literature as well as from clinical observation and patient reports.

- **Local or systemic events that cause hyperemia to the tissues of the involved limb(s):** Examples include hot packs to the involved limb, hot tubs, summer weather, handling hot foods directly, aggressive massage, overuse of the involved limb, infection, soft tissue sprains, and/or strains. Muscle exertion, especially vigorous types, produces microtrauma to tissues surrounding the involved joints. This may in turn lead to localized inflammation, hyperemia, and swelling. In the individual with a normal lymphatic system, this is resolved by the body without any lasting effects. In the individual with a limb at risk, it may be the final imbalance that tilts the scale and results in lymphedema or exacerbates a subclinical case. For further discussion on the effects of exercise on the lymphatic system, refer to Chapter 4.
- **Changes in pressure:** Examples include airplane travel, which involves pressure changes that allow interstitial fluid to pool in the dependent extremities while the vasomotor activity of the lymphangion is at a low level (the individual is at rest during the flight).[34] Lowered cabin pressure in aircraft may further exacerbate an already incompetent lymphatic system, causing the initial visible symptoms of a new or existing but subclinical case of lymphedema.[35] While swimming is a beneficial exercise, scuba diving has been reported as a trigger for the onset of signs and symptoms of lymphedema. The significant decrease in hydrostatic pressure upon return to the surface may be the source of the problem. Pressure changes alter the ability of the system to regulate fluid hydrostatic pressure and may cause a flood of fluid into an already incompetent system. Changes in pressure can also refer to any other external applications of pressure that affect local hydrostatic pressure and have the potential to be the stimulus for onset of symptoms. Examples would include prolonged wear of tight fitting clothing over areas at risk, use of aggressive massage techniques to the area at risk, or sleeping for long periods of time on the limb at risk.
- **Insult to skin integrity:** In keeping with evidence that infection is a risk factor for developing lymphedema, examples of triggers representing a few of many possible incidents that could serve as stimuli for the onset of the signs and symptoms include: pet scratches, gardening related injuries, insect bites, contusions, injections, or intravenous cannulation[36].
- **Changes in weight and body fluid volumes:** Examples may include pregnancy, weight gain, chronic venous insufficiency, related complications from other health problems, and certain medications.

CLINICAL DIAGNOSIS

The diagnosis of lymphedema is usually straightforward and can be made in the clinic without the use of specialized tests. The most useful information will be derived from a thorough patient history, systems review, and tests and measurements including inspection and palpation. Differential diagnosis should also be part of the examination process. Examples of what to include in the examination are shown in Chapter 3. You may also want to refer back to the morphological progression outlined in Chapter 1.

Some referring practitioners and clinicians deem it important to *grade* or *stage* the lymphedema before treatment begins. Establishing a level of severity may be useful in predicting length of intervention, or for comparisons in collection of adherence, quality of life, and clinical outcomes data. *Grading or staging, however, is not universally used or understood by referring practitioners or other health professionals and should be accompanied by documentation of additional objective information in the examination results.* Four commonly used staging scales are included here.

REVIEW OF PITTING RESPONSE

Pitting occurs when pressure is applied to a specific spot with the examiner's finger and an indentation remains. The implication is that the onset of swelling is more recent and, by some examiners' estimates, less serious. A nonpitting response occurs when pressure applied to a specific spot does not leave a noticeable indentation. The implication is that swelling is significant, more advanced fibrotic changes have occurred subcutaneously, and fluid cannot be displaced with mere pressure.

INTERNATIONAL SOCIETY OF LYMPHOLOGY (ISL) CLASSIFICATION SYSTEM—1985[37]

Grade 1   Pits on pressure; largely or completely reduced with elevation; slight or no clinical fibrosis.

Grade 2   Nonpitting on pressure; not reduced with elevation; moderate to severe clinical fibrosis.

Elephantiasis Signs and symptoms of elephantiasis may be present in Grade 2 but because it varies greatly among patients, a subclassification with five categories has been added.[38]

STAGES OF LYMPHEDEMA

Subclinical   Patient begins to feel "heaviness" in limb, fibrotic changes and fluid accumulation can occur before visible swelling or pitting. Approximately 50% of patients with minimal edema report a feeling of heaviness or fullness in the extremity.[4]

Stage I   Reversible lymphedema: accumulation of protein-rich fluid, elevation reduces swelling. Pits on pressure.

Stage II   Spontaneously irreversible lymphedema: proteins stimulate fibroblast formation, connective and scar tissue proliferate. Minimal pitting even with moderate swelling.

Stage III   Lymphostatic elephantiasis: hardening of dermal tissues, papillomas of the skin, appearance elephant-like. (Not everyone progresses to this stage.)

―――――

Dr. Michael Földi, 1985

CLASSIFICATION FOR EDEMA[a]

Edema is not detectable clinically until interstitial volume reaches 30% above normal.

1+   Edema that is barely detectable

2+   A slight indentation is visible when the skin is depressed. (*Author's note:* A slight indentation remains *following* skin depression.)

3+   A deeper fingerprint returns to normal in 5 to 30 seconds.

4+   The extremity may be 1.5 to 2 times normal size.

―――――

[a]Classic scale known to most physicians

CLASSIFICATION FOR LYMPHEDEMA[39]

Mild[b]   Less than 3 centimeters (cm) differential between affected limb and unaffected limb.

Moderate   3 to 5 cm differential between affected limb and unaffected limb.

Severe   5+ cm differential between affected limb and unaffected limb.

―――――

[b]There is some concern among management experts that this classification scale may not represent the patient's condition adequately. The size differential between limbs does not indicate the length of time since onset of fluid accumulation (before it was visible), how long measurable swelling has been present, the amount of tissue fibrosis that has occurred, or the presence of palpable tissue resistance. While a smaller limb may indicate fewer functional limitations, it does not always correlate with level of severity, level of discomfort, cosmetic acceptance, or quality of life. To determine frequency of visits and duration of the episode of care based on a centimeter differential between limbs implies that a smaller limb is not as involved clinically as a larger limb. While it is likely that the larger differentials represent a more severe condition, the reverse is not always true. In light of mounting interest in the possible link between early posttherapeutic swelling and the ultimate development of lymphedema, it is prudent to suspect that some patients with smaller limb differentials may present with more involved signs and symptoms than the measurements imply.

OTHER DIAGNOSTIC TESTS

A thorough physical examination is felt to be the gold standard for the diagnosis of lymphedema.[40] When there is doubt regarding a clinical diagnosis, the following diagnostic tests may be helpful. The use of imaging methods for diagnosis, however, is usually only necessary if exact morphological information is needed, when a combined form of lymphedema is suspected, or for research purposes. Infrequently, imaging techniques are used to determine treatment and assess the therapeutic response to treatment.[41]

Lymphangiography—An oily contrast medium is injected into a lymphatic vessel in the foot or hand. Serial x-rays are taken of the limb. Movement of the tracer is studied. Lymph collectors can be demonstrated. The procedure has considerable morbidity.[3] Occasionally individuals react to the contrast medium causing inflammation and

FIGURE 2-1 Pelvic and Abdominal Lymph Nodes and Lymphatics Visualized by Lymphangiography

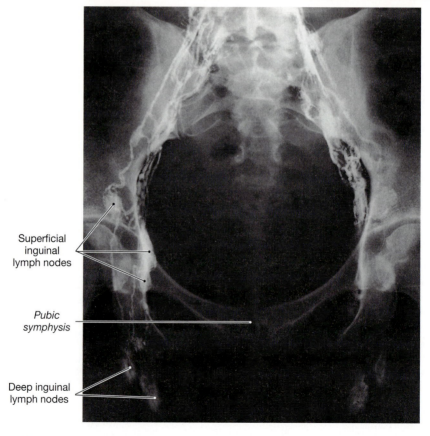

Superficial inguinal lymph nodes

Pubic symphysis

Deep inguinal lymph nodes

(Courtesy of *Human Anatomy, 3/e* by Martini/Timmons/McKinley© 2000. Reprinted by permission of Pearson Education, Inc., Upper Saddle River, NJ.)

FIGURE 2-2 Example of Child with Primary Lymphedema

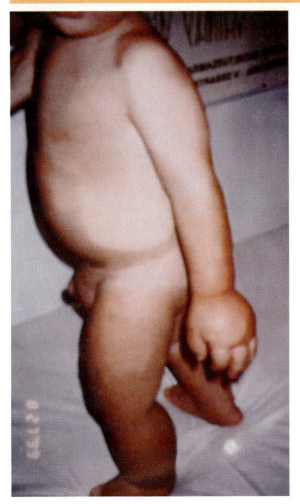

(Courtesy of Klose Norton Training & Consulting, LLC)

subsequent blockage of the lymphatic. This reaction can contribute to further impairment of the lymphatic system.

Fluorescent microlymphography—A subepidermal injection of a fluorescent tracer
is used, often near the medial malleolus. A fluorescent microscope and a video camera record diffusion of the fluorescent substance. Many lymph system functions can be
observed. Superficial cutaneous lymph capillaries can be imaged.

Lymphoscintigraphy (or lymphangioscintigraphy–LAS)—A radioactive substance is
injected into the back of the hand or foot. A gamma camera and computer are used to
observe a wide variety of lymph system functions including but not limited to rate of
lymph fluid movement and lymph node uptake speeds. There has been no reported
morbidity associated with this procedure.[4]

FIGURE 2-3 Example of Secondary Lymphedema of the Upper Extremity following Breast Cancer Treatment.

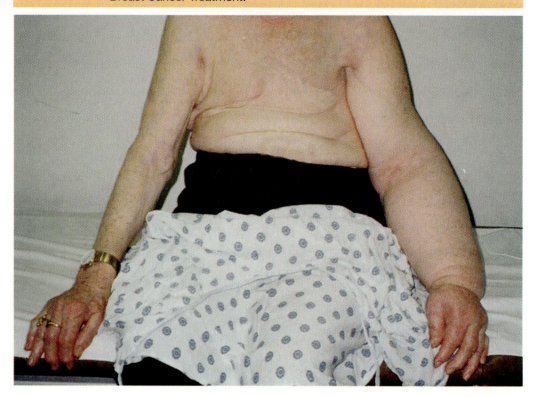

(Courtesy of Deborah G. Kelly)

Computed tomography (CT)—radiological imaging providing cross-sectional views. Application is limited to identification of secondary lymphedema due to malignancy.

Magnetic Resonance Imaging (MRI)—Noninvasive imaging method obtained without the use of radiation by placing the body in a magnetic field. In contradistinction to LAS (page 39), MRI can visualize lymph trunks, nodes, and soft tissues proximal to sites of lymphatic obstruction. Results especially useful when combined with LAS.[43]

Ultrasound—The velocity of high-frequency sound waves through body tissues is measured. Limited mainly to the identification of lymphoceles and lymphangiomas. It can also reveal adult filaria in preparation for surgical removal.

Duplex Ultrasound Scan—Color and gray scale imaging are used with Doppler ultrasound assessment of blood flow. Venous outflow and arterial inflow can be measured. The possibility of venous and arterial components to the lymphedema can be assessed.[44]

FIGURE 2-4 Example of Secondary Lymphedema of the Lower Legs Caused by Filariasis

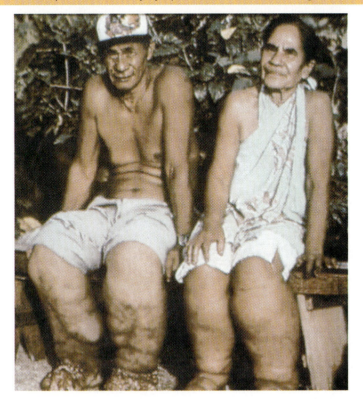

(Courtesy of Klose Norton Training & Consulting, LLC)

FIGURE 2-5 Example of Primary Lymphedema (Tarda) of the Lower Extremity Triggered by an Ankle Sprain.

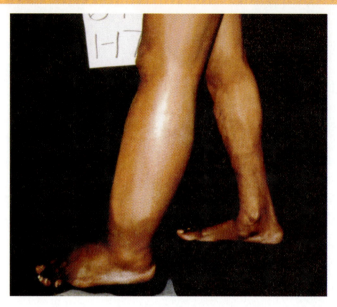

(Courtesy of Guthrie Healthcare System: Guthrie Lymphedema Clinic)

FIGURE 2-6 Example of Primary Lymphedema, Bilateral Lower Extremities, with Lymphostatic Elephantiasis, Triggering Event Unknown.

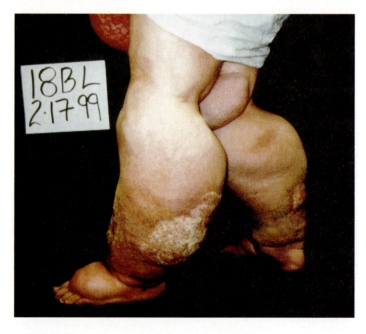

(Courtesy of Guthrie Healthcare System: Guthrie Lymphedema Clinic)

References

1. Földi, E., Földi, M., Clodius, L. 1989. The lymphedema chaos: A lancet. *Ann Plast Surg.* 22:505–15.
2. Szuba, A. and Rockson, S.G. 1997. Lymphedema: Anatomy, physiology and pathogenesis. *Vascular Medicine* 2:321–26.
3. Casley-Smith, J.R. and Casley-Smith, J.R. 1994. *Modern Treatment for Lymphoedema.* The Lymphoedema Association of Australia, Inc., University of Adelaide, SA 5005, Australia.
4. Brennan, M.J. 1992. Lymphedema following the surgical treatment of breast cancer: A review of pathophysiology and treatment. *Journal of Pain and Symptom Management* 7 (2):110–16.
5. Casley-Smith, J. R. 1995. Alterations of untreated lymphedema and its grades over time. *Lymphology* 28(4):174–85.
6. Daane, S., Poltoratszy, P., Rockwell, W. B. 1998. Postmastectomy lymphedema management: Evolution of the complex decongestive therapy technique. *Ann Plast Surg.* 40:128–34.
7. DeLisa, J. A. 1993. *Rehabilitation Medicine: Principles and Practice,* 2nd ed. Philadelphia: Lippincott.
8. Weissleder, H. and Schuchhardt, C. 1997. *Lymphedema, Diagnosis and Therapy*, 2nd ed. Bonn: Kagerer Kommunication.
9. Petereit, D. G., Mehta, M. P., Buchler, D. A., Kinsella, T. J. 1993. A retrospective review of nodal treatment for vulvar cancer. *Am J Clin Oncol.* 16(1):38–42.
10. Werngren-Elgstrom, M. and Lidman D. 1994. Lymphoedema of the lower extremities after surgery and radiotherapy for cancer of the cervix. *Scand J Plast Reconstr Hand Surg.* 28:289–93.
11. Kavoussi, L., Sosa, E., Chandhoke, P., Chodak, G., et al. 1993. Complications of laparoscopic pelvic lymph node dissection. *J Urol.* 149:322–25.
12. Ko, D., Lerner, R., Klose, G., Cosimi, A. 1998. Effective treatment of lymphedema of the extremities. *Arch Surg.* 133:452–58.
13. Karakousis, C., Heiser, M., Moore, R. 1983. Lymphedema after groin dissection. *Am J Surg.* 145:205–08.
14. Wrone, D., Tanabe, K., Cosimi, A., Gadd, M., Souba, W., Sober, A. 2000. Lymphedema after sentinel lymph node dissection biopsy for cutaneous melanoma. *Arch Dermatol.* 136:511–14.
15. Martimbeau, P., Kjorstad, K., Kolstad, P. 1978. Stage 1B carcinoma of the cervix, the Norwegian Radium Hospital, 1968–1970. Results of treatment and major complications. *Am J Obstet Gynecol.* 131:389–94.
16. Rotmensch, J., Rubin, S., Sutton, H., Javaheri, G., et al. 1990. Preoperative radiotherapy followed by radical vulvectomy with inguinal lymphadenectomy for advanced vulvar carcinoma. *Gynecol Oncol.* 36:181–84.
17. Bognar, J., Nagy, P., Kadar, E., Bajtal, A., Mayer, A., Daroczy, J., Jakab, F. 1997. The current surgical treatment of primary malignant melanoma of the skin. *Acta Chir Hung.* 36:37–38.
18. Földi, M. 1998. Are there enigmas concerning the pathophysiology of lymphedema after breast cancer treatment? *NLN Newsletter* 10(4):1–4.
19. Kissin, M. W., Querci della Rovere, G., Easton, D., Westbury, G. 1986. Risk of lymphoedema following the treatment of breast cancer. *Br J Surg.* 73:580–84.
20. Yeoh, E. K., Denham, J. W., Davies, S. A., Spittle, M. F. 1986. Primary breast cancer. Complications of axillary management. *Acta Radiol Oncol.* 25:105–08.
21. Aitken, R. J., Gaze, M. N., Rodger, A., et al. 1989. Arm morbidity within a trial of mastectomy and either nodal sample with selective radiotherapy or axillary clearance. *Br J Surg.* 76:569–71.
22. Dewar, J. A., Sarrazin, D., Benhamou, E., et al. 1987. Management of the axilla in conservatively treated breast cancer: 592 patients treated at Institut Gustave-Roussy. *Int J Radiat Oncol Biol Phys.* 13:475–81.
23. Tsyb, A. F., Bardychev, M. S., Guseve, L. I. 1981. Secondary limb edema following irradiation. *Lymphology* 14:127–32.
24. Aitken, D. and Minton, J. P. 1983. Complications associated with mastectomy. *Surg Clin North Am.* 63:1331–52.
25. Mortimer, P. S. 2000. Implications of the lymphatic system in CVI-associated edema. *Angiology* 51:3–7.

26. Ramelet, A. A. 2000. Pharmacologic aspects of a phlebotropic drug in CVI-associated edema. *Angiology* 51:19–23.

27. Rockson, S. G. 1998. Precipitating factors in lymphedema: Myths and realities. *Cancer* 83(S12B):2814-16.

28. Segerstrom, K., Bjerle, P., Graffman, S., Nystrom, A. 1992. Factors that influence the incidence of brachial oedema after treatment of breast cancer. *Scan J Plast Reconstr Surg Hand Surg.* 26:223–27.

29. Kissin, M., Querci della Rovere, G., Easton, D., Westbury, G. 1986. Risk of lymphedema following the treatment of breast cancer. *Br J Surg.* 73:580–84.

30. Casley-Smith, J. 1995. Alterations of untreated lymphedema and its grades over time. *Lymphology* 28:174–85.

31. Ryan, T. J. and Curri, S. B. 1989. The microcirculation of fat in man: The importance of the regulation of blood flow. *Clinics in Dermatology* 7:25–36.

32. Petrek, J. A. *News from MSKCC: Cancer News: June 1998. www.mskcc.org.*

33. Tunkel, R. S. and Lachmann E. 1998. Lymphedema of the limb: An overview of treatment options. *Postgraduate Medicine* 104:131–44.

34. Schuch, W. J. 1998. In defense of the 18 steps to prevention. *NLN Newsletter.* 10(4):6–7.

35. Casley-Smith, J. and Casley-Smith, J. 1996. Lymphedema initiated by aircraft flights. *Aviat Space Environ Med.* 67:52–56.

36. Smith, J. 1998. The practice of venepuncture in lymphoedema. *European Journal of Cancer Care* 7:97–98.

37. Casley-Smith, J. R., Foldi, M., Ryan, T. J., et al. 1985. Lymphedema: Summary of the 10th International Congress of Lymphology Working Group discussions and recommendations. Adelaide, Australia, August 10–17, 1985. *Lymphology* 18:175–80.

38. Casley-Smith, J. R. and Casley-Smith, J.R. 1994. *Modern Treatment for Lymphedema.* The Lymphedema Association of Australia, Inc. p 88.

39. APTA. 2001. Guide to physical therapist practice. *Phys Ther.* 8(1):21–746.

40. Rockson, S. et al. 1998. Workgroup III: Diagnosis and management of lymphedema. *Cancer* (Supplement) 83(12):2882–85.

41. Bourgeois, P., Leduc, O., Leduc, A. 1998. Imaging techniques in the management and prevention of posttherapeutic upper limb edemas. *Cancer* (Supplement) 83: 2805–13.

42. Case, T. C., Witte, C. L., Witte, M. H., Unger, E. C., Williams, W. H. 1992. Magnetic resonance imaging in human lymphedema: Comparison with lymphangioscintigraphy. *Magnetic Resonance Imaging* 10:549–58.

43. Svensson, W. E., Mortimer, P. S., Tohno, E., Cosgrove, D.O. 1994. Increased arterial inflow demonstrated by Doppler ultrasound in arm swelling following breast cancer treatment. *Eur J Cancer* 30A(5):661–64.

3

PATIENT MANAGEMENT

It is important that health care workers have a high index of suspicion about lymphedema, as treatment is easier when initiated in the early, milder stages of the condition.

DR. RICHARD TUNKEL

INTRODUCTION

The first interaction between the health care provider and the patient with lymphedema or a limb at risk will be the beginning of an intense, possibly lengthy, professional relationship. The precision of the examination, the clarity of the documentation, and the effectiveness of the intervention will be important to the patient, the clinician, the insurance provider, and other disciplines involved in the care of this person.

There is now movement toward facilitation of communication among medical professionals worldwide. Adoption of a uniform definition of terms and a shift in the type of model used is important to the exchange of ideas and scientific findings. The intent is to "establish a common language for describing functional status associated with health conditions."[1] There are several models or combinations of models being utilized by health care professionals to make the transition. The move is from the *medical model*, which was strictly diagnosis based, to the *sociomedical model*, which gives a broader picture to describe health status. Names you may see in the literature will include the ICIDH,[2] the ICIDH-Beta 2,[2] Nagi's Model of Disability,[3] and Verbrugge and Jette's Disablement Process Model.[4] All of these have been valuable in shaping the way patient management is viewed. Schenkman states that "using disablement models encourages clinicians to encompass a more global view of problem solving and to incorporate preventive strategies at the earliest stage of the disablement process."[5]

Any health care professional or student reading this chapter will benefit from the use of a format that is sensitive to the changing atmosphere and trends in terminology and philosophy for managing patients/clients. Today's health professional should be positioned on the leading edge of this rapid movement toward universal, common terminology and the philosophy that disability is a sociomedical concept.

It is imperative that before the referral process begins, all potential referring practitioners (M.D., P.A., A.R.N.P., D.M.D., D.D.S.) are provided with appropriate information regarding all possible systems of involvement when lymphedema is present. This can be accomplished in a variety of means but examples might include: additions to professional curriculi; inservices; textbooks; special interest study groups; and informational letters to group practices or individual practitioners. The patient should receive optimal management including thorough assessment of associated dysfunctions that frequently accompany the symptoms of lymphedema. *If the intervention is too narrowly focused, it is unlikely to be as effective as a more comprehensive approach.*

Following referral, or self-referral in regions with Direct Access,[a] the health care provider will begin the patient relationship by addressing elements of management. The remainder of the chapter includes a suggested scheme of management that reflects the changes mentioned in the introduction to this chapter. The scheme has been adapted from the *Guide to Physical Therapist Practice.*[6] This process illustrates the application of disablement models in managing the patient with lymphedema. Specific references to physical therapy have been omitted to demonstrate the *universality* of the concepts.

ELEMENTS OF PATIENT MANAGEMENT

I. Examination
   A. History
   B. Systems review
   C. Tests and measurements
II. Evaluation
   A. Diagnosis
   B. Prognosis
III. Intervention
   A. Coordination, communication, documentation
   B. Patient-related instruction
   C. Direct intervention

EXAMINATION

The examination is like an *investigation.* There are three components to the examination: *history, relevant systems reviews,* and any appropriate *tests and measurements.*

History: The history will be essential for correct identification of lymphedema. In addition to general demographics, social history, occupation, and environmental information, the following is important information to solicit:

- Onset of symptoms, identification of the triggering event.
- Length of time since initial onset of symptoms.
- Past and current health status, medical and surgical history: Identify what initial disease, insult, or event damaged a component of the lymphatic system. This will be the point at which you identify and document the existence of a *limb(s) at risk* or the possibility of subclinical lymphedema.
- Presence or absence of pain and to what degree: If pain is significant, this may suggest the need for tests and measures to determine if pain is from a secondary problem.
- Health risk factors, co-existing health problems, family history: This information will be especially important when primary lymphedema is

---

[a]Direct Access is the ability to treat patients without the legal requirements of a physician or other practitioner referral.

suspected. It will also be useful since the presence of other health problems (comorbidities) may complicate recovery.

- Medications: Some play a role in recovery, others may delay healing.
- Functional status and activity level: Include social habits that may affect your intervention such as smoking, level of physical fitness, and weight management.
- Review of available records, including lab tests, diagnostic tests.
- Past intervention for the symptoms: It will be important to know what other interventions have been applied since some of them may have led to exacerbation of the signs and symptoms.

Some of this information could be collected in the form of a questionnaire to be filled in by the patient before or during the first visit. Compilation of additional data is needed to further understand precipitating events or *triggers,* which mark the onset of the signs and symptoms of lymphedema.

Systems Review: A brief systems review will provide additional information about the general health of the patient. This will help you to identify possible health problems that require consultation with another health care provider. Information gathered from a systems review may affect decisions about which examination procedures to use and how the intervention plan will be designed. Each individual systems review will differ according to the unique signs and symptoms revealed. Because this is a brief review, documentation might indicate "impaired" versus "not impaired" for each example. It is important to collect data on the status of the following systems:

- *Cardiopulmonary:* B/P, pulse, respiratory rate
- *Integumentary:* initially brief, later extensive look at texture, color, integrity, tension
- *Musculoskeletal:* gross findings of symmetry, range of motion and strength
- *Neuromuscular:* gait, mobility, balance, motor control
- *Communication ability:* affect, cognition, language, and learning style

Tests and Measurements: The patient is examined more specifically at this time with tests and measures that elicit additional information. State Practice Acts and scope of practice should dictate who performs and interprets the results of the tests and measurements. It is crucial that referring practitioners are provided with appropriate educational material regarding all possible systems of involvement where lymphedema is present. This will assure that adequate intervention for the signs and symptoms of lymphedema is planned and, also, that the patient will receive optimal intervention for associated dysfunctions that may accompany the presence of lymphedema. Potential associated dysfunctions are unique to the individual but could include examples such as posture and gait deviations, strength and conditioning deficits, and/or difficulties with activities of daily living. The decision about which tests and measurements to use and how many will be based on the complexity of the condition and other information derived from the history and the systems review. During the examination, additional problems may be identified and specific tests and measurements may be required to sufficiently make an evaluation, establish a diagnosis and a prognosis, and select interventions.

Tests and measurements that may be included for a patient with lymphedema or one at risk of developing lymphedema are arranged here in order of importance:[7] The purpose of this compilation is to alert the reader to the tests and measurements. It is assumed that both students and experienced clinicians will utilize the education received within their disciplines to perform appropriate tests and measurements or will refer to the most qualified professional to conduct the examination.

- **Integumentary integrity:** Extensive *palpation and inspection* are of utmost importance in determining level of severity and the subsequent intervention plan. Included in this category will be texture, color, pitting status, fibrosis, temperature, and presence of cysts/fistulas, papillomas, or ulcerations. Staging or grading can be done as appropriate at this time. (See Chapter 2 for staging and grading scales.) Physical evidence of subclinical lymphedema may be obtained at this point. The *Stemmer's skin fold test* can provide additional information. When thickened skin folds at the base of the second toe or second finger are resistant to lifting, a *positive Stemmer's sign* is noted. A negative skin fold test, however, does not exclude lymphedema.

- **Anthropometric characteristics:** Included in this category are volumetric and/or circumferential measurements. Some clinicians use a mathematical formula for cone volume[8,9] to further describe limb volumes. An additional examination measurement uses the *tonometer*.[10,11] Soft-tissue tonometry uses a tension-measuring device that presses on the skin. The greater the tension reading, the less compliant the skin, implying the presence of fluid and/or fibrosis. Tonometry is useful for determining subclinical evidence of lymphedema as changes can be detected and measured before circumferential or volumetric changes are seen. This is not yet a standardized procedure. *Bioelectrical impedance analysis* is showing great promise at providing accurate measures of lymphedema and in predicting early onset of lymphedema before clinical diagnosis is possible.[12]

- **Joint integrity and mobility, Muscle performance, Range of motion, Posture:** Manual muscle tests, goniometry, and isokinetic tools are current standards for measurement. Many patients with lymphedema will present with significant limitations in these four categories.

- **Pain:** There are numerous scales for measuring pain. A Visual Analog Scale (VAS) is adequate for this type of patient examination. The location of the pain will be of utmost importance in determining if the pain is related to the lymphedema or is related to another problem.

- **Arousal, mentation, cognition:** Since much of the success of the intervention will be contingent upon the patient's level of involvement, it is important to assess the patient's ability to understand the treatment protocol and follow instructions.

- **Ventilation, respiration, and circulation:** This includes the vascular exam and venous patterns that might contribute to the function of the lymphatic system. If lower extremity involvement is present, and the *systems review* and *differential diagnosis* indicate the potential for circulatory disorders, it is appropriate to seek assessment of the circulation using the *Ankle Brachial Index (ABI)*. The ABI is a noninvasive assessment of circulation. It is a *comparative* assessment of peripheral to more central blood pressure that gives an idea of arterial patency/sufficiency. A handheld Doppler ultrasound is used to make the assessment. An ABI value is a calculated value. A value of <0.8 or lower implies that arterial circulation is insufficient. Clinically, the implication is that compression is contraindicated. A manual palpation/screening of the abdominal region is appropriate to determine patient tolerance to the deep breathing and resisted breathing portions of the manual therapy performed during the treatment phase.

- **Sensory and reflex integrity:** These tests are particularly important when signs and symptoms are long-standing, the individual complains of numbness or tingling in the affected limb, or when the individual also has a diagnosis of diabetes or a circulatory disorder.
- **Motor function, Gait, locomotion, and balance:** These issues are especially important with lower extremity involvement but can be affected with severe upper extremity involvement. If neglected during the examination, the person's ability to regain optimal levels of function may be hindered. The exercise portion of the intervention plan may also be limited by lack of function in this category.
- **Orthotic, protective, and supportive devices:** The need for these is particularly important with lower extremity involvement but can be affected with upper extremity involvement as well.
- **Assistive and adaptive devices:** Assessing a person's need for such devices should be included in the examination. Appropriate professional collaboration should be sought if the individual performing the examination is not skilled in this type of assessment.
- **Aerobic capacity and endurance:** Due to the importance of exercise during the treatment phase and the self-management phase, basic measurements should be taken so that an appropriate exercise program can be designed. The *BORG Scale of Perceived Exertion* would be an example of an appropriate tool for this category.[13]
- **Self-care and home management:** During the initial examination, the person's ability to manage the challenges of the intensive intervention program must be assessed. Alterations to the intervention plan will be based largely on the person's ability or lack of ability to participate in the self-management portion of the treatment.
- **Community and work integration or reintegration, environmental, home, and work barriers:** If not assessed at the initial examination, these issues must be addressed by the end of the treatment phase and before the self-management phase begins. Depending on the level of severity of the lymphedema, the return to work and home can imply major adjustments and changes for the patient and the involved family members.

EVALUATION

The evaluation is the process of using *clinical judgment* to make decisions. It can also be called the process of *clinical decision making*. Historically, the *evaluation* has been identified as the *assessment*. You may know it as the "A" portion of a SOAP note. The change in terminology better reflects the professional judgment required to process information gained during the examination in order to make clinical decisions about diagnosis, prognosis, and intervention. Health care providers make judgments concerning the patient. These judgments should be based on the clinical findings, extent of loss of function, social considerations, and the patient's overall physical function and health status. The evaluation process sets the course for reducing impairment, functional limitation, and disability. It should reflect:[7]

- chronicity or severity of the problem
- possibility of multisite or multisystem involvement
- presence of preexisting systemic conditions or diseases
- stability of the condition

  Appropriate health care providers should also consider:

- level of current impairments
- probability of prolonged impairment
- functional limitation and disability
- living environment
- potential discharge destinations
- social supports

Diagnosis

The diagnosis will describe a *cluster of signs and symptoms.* The diagnostic process includes looking at the information from the examination, organizing it into clusters, and interpreting it. The diagnosis will guide the health care provider in determining the most appropriate intervention strategy for the patient. The diagnostic process often includes collaboration with other health professionals, sharing findings, and including other referral sources to ensure optimal care. In regions with Direct Access, if the patient presents to you as their entry into the system, it is advisable that a physician be immediately consulted to become part of the treatment team. The complexity of lymphedema and the potential for confounding factors make physician involvement important. **Thoughtful and thorough differential diagnosis should occur at this time in the examination process.** There are other diagnoses that may appear clinically like lymphedema but are not lymphedema. What is more likely is that lymphedema is present in addition to another diagnosis. The combined effects of two or more pathologies may render the patient considerably more involved. Realistic goals and predicted outcomes must be considered when several pathologies are noted. Listed below are examples of diagnoses that should be ruled out before intervention begins:

- deep vein thrombosis
- muscle trauma
- malignancy
- CRPS—Chronic Regional Pain Syndrome (Historically known as RSD-Reflex Sympathetic Dystrophy)
- Cor pulmonale—Right-sided heart failure, and left-sided heart failure with pulmonary edema (the general term *congestive heart failure* (CHF) is sometimes used but is less accurate and descriptive)

- kidney disease
- chronic venous insufficiency (CVI)[14,15]

If lymphedema coexists with these diagnoses, it can often be treated successfully. Close communication with the referring practitioner and other medical professionals will be essential.

Prognosis

The prognosis provides information about the predicted level of improvement in function for the patient. It also includes a *prediction* about the amount of time needed to reach the optimal level of function. Now, the health care provider establishes a plan of care. The plan of care should include:

- anticipated goals and expected outcomes (formerly referred to as short-term and long-term goals)
- specific interventions to be used
- duration and frequency of intervention
- criteria for discharge

INTERVENTION

The intervention is the actual skilled interaction of the health professional with the patient and other individuals involved in patient care. There are three components to intervention:

Coordination, communication, and documentation represent the first component. These describe services that should be provided for all patients during the course of their treatment. Services may include coordination of care with all involved parties, appropriate documentation, education, record reviews, discharge planning, and referrals to other resources. This will be very important for the patient with lymphedema who often has multisystem involvement and a complicated history with several involved health care providers. Patients can benefit from support groups, counseling, additional reading materials, and Internet access.

Patient-related instruction will be crucial to the long-term success of the intervention plan for patients with lymphedema or a limb at risk. Lymphedema is a chronic condition that requires diligent follow-up by the patient and family or other involved parties. Much of the success of the treatment phase and its potential for lasting results will be based on the adherence of the patient to the program during the self-management phase. It is essential that patients understand what to do and what their role is in their symptom management. Instruction will be most valuable if presented in a variety of forms: Health care providers should strive for clarity, quality, and attention to educational background of the audience in their instructional materials. Examples might include:

- *Audio-visuals:* video tapes or computer programs showing exercises and bandaging (purchased or made on site)
- *Written instructions* on prevention and control, exercise, skin care. (See sample in Chapter 8, which can be copied and distributed to patients.)
- *Verbal and written demonstrations* of bandaging and exercise
- *Literature:* books and articles on coping with lymphedema

Direct intervention will be selected, applied, or modified by the appropriate health care provider based on the results of all components of the management scheme: examination, evaluation, diagnosis, prognosis—goals and outcomes. Reexamination may be necessary based on the results of the intervention. Following reexamination, a different intervention may be appropriate. Referral to another professional or discontinuation of care may result. *Because of the variety of interventions currently promoted for lymphedema, and the failure of historical treatments to provide long lasting effects, a clinician who does not see positive results with a given intervention would be advised to seek additional professional input before deciding on discontinuation of care.*

The next section represents an example of a template that could be used for a patient with lymphedema during the initial visit. This form follows the principles of universal terminology and the sociomedical model described at the beginning of this chapter. The design loosely follows a template suggested by the American Physical Therapy Association.[b] Revisions have been made to demonstrate the universality of the principles and to create a form applicable for all health practitioners.

References

1. International Classification of Functioning and Disabilitiy-Beta 2 Draft, Full Version July 1999, World Health Organization, Geneva, Switzerland (ICIDH-2) p 9.
2. International Classification of Impairments, Disabilities and Handicaps. 1994. World Health Organization, Geneva, Switzerland (ICIDH).
3. Nagi, S. 1969. *Disability and Rehabilitation.* Columbus, OH: Ohio State University Press.
4. Verbrugge, L. M. and Jette, A. M. 1994. The disablement process. *Soc Sci Med.* (Jan)38(1):1–14.
5. Schenkman, M., et al. 1999. Multisystem model for management of neurologically impaired adults—An update and illustrative case. *Neurology Report* 23(4):145–57.
6. Guide to physical therapist practice. 1997. *Phys Ther.* 77(11):1163-1650.
7. This list has been adapted from *Model Definition of Physical Therapy for State Practice Acts.* Guide to Physical Therapist Practice. *Phys Ther.* 1997;77(11):1178.
8. Casley-Smith, J. R. and Casley-Smith, J. R.

1994. *Modern Treatment for Lymphoedema.* Lymphoedema Assoc. Australia, Uni. Adel., S.A. 5005, Australia, pp.90–112.
9. Casley-Smith, J. R. 1994. Measuring and representing peripheral oedema and its alterations. *Lymphology* 27:56–70.
10. Clodius, L., Deak, L., Piller, N. B. 1976. A new instrument for evaluation of tissue tonicity in lymphedema. *Lymphology* 9:1–5.
11. Chen, H. C., O'Brien, B., Pribaz, J.J., Roberts, A.H.N. 1988. The use of tonometry in the assessment of upper extremity lymphedema. *Br J Plast Surg.* 41:399–402.
12. Cornish, B. H., et al. 2000. Early diagnosis of lymphedema in postsurgery breast cancer patients. *Ann N Y Acad Sci.* 904:571–74.
13. Borg, G. A. 1982. Psychophysical bases of perceived exertion. *Med Sci Sports Exerc.* 14(5):377–81.
14. Mortimer, P. S. 2000. Implications of the lymphatic system in CVI-associated edema. *Angiology* 51:3–7.
15. Ramelet, A. A. 2000. Pharmacologic aspect of a phlebotropic drug in CVI-associated edema. *Angiology* 51:19–23.

[b]Adapted from Appendix 6: Documentation Template, *Guide to Physical Therapist Practice* 2nd Edition, pp 707–719 with permission from the American Physical Therapy Association.

Patient/Client Management
Outpatient: LYMPHEDEMA

Date: _____

Patient ID#: _____

IDENTIFICATION INFORMATION

Name:

_____
Last

_____
First   **MI**

	Month	**Day**	**Year**
Date of Birth:	☐☐	☐☐	☐☐

Sex: ☐ Male   ☐ Female

Dominant Hand: ☐ Right   ☐ Left   ☐ Unknown

Race	**Ethnicity**	**Language**
☐ Asian	☐ Hispanic/Latino	☐ English understood
☐ Black		☐ Interpreter needed?
☐ White	Primary language: _____	

Referred by: _____

Recent medical hx & reason for referral:_____

DEMOGRAPHIC INFORMATION

Cultural/Religious

Any customs or religious beliefs or wishes that might affect care?

_____
_____
_____

Education:
Highest grade completed (circle one): 1 2 3 4 5 6 7 8 9 10 11 12

☐ Some college/technical school
☐ College graduate
☐ Graduate school/advanced degree

Employment:

☐ Working full-time outside home   ☐ Homemaker
☐ Working full-time from home   ☐ Student
☐ Working part-time outside home   ☐ Retired
☐ Working part-time from home   ☐ Unemployed

Occupation:_____

Has patient completed an advanced directive?
☐ Yes   ☐ No

PATIENT RESOURCES

Type of Residence:

☐ Private home
☐ Private apartment
☐ Rented room
☐ Board & care/assisted living/group home
☐ Homeless (with or without shelter)
☐ Long-term care facility (nursing home)
☐ Hospice
☐ Unknown
☐ Other

Lives with:

☐ Alone
☐ Spouse/significant other only
☐ Spouse/significant other(s)
☐ Child (not spouse)
☐ Other relative(s) (not spouse or children)
☐ Group setting
☐ Personal care attendant
☐ Unknown
☐ Other

Environment:

☐ Stairs, no railing
☐ Stairs, railing
☐ Ramps
☐ Elevator
☐ Uneven terrain
☐ Other obstacles: _____

Caregiver status:
Presence of family member/friend willing & able to assist patient?
☐ Yes   ☐ No

Past use of community services: 0=No 1=Unknown 2=Yes
Day services/programs	Mental health services ☐
Home health services	Respiratory therapy ☐
Homemaking services	"Therapies (PT,OT,SLP)" ☐
Hospice	Other (eg: volunteer): _____
Meals on Wheels	_____

Available social supports: 0=No 1=Possibly Yes 2=Definitely

☐ Emotional support
☐ Intermittent physical support with ADLs or IADLs (less than daily)
☐ Intermittent physical support with ADLs or IADLs—daily
☐ Full-time physical support (as needed)
☐ All or most of necessary transportation

Lymphedema Examination

PATIENT HISTORY

General Health

a. Patient rates health as:

☐ Excellent ☐ Good ☐ Fair ☐ Poor

b. Major life changes during the past year?

☐ No ☐ Yes

Height: _____

Weight: _____

Has weight changed in the last year?

☐ Yes ☐ No

Comments: _____

_____

_____

Health Habits:

a. Exercise

(1) Exercises beyond normal daily activities and chores?

☐ No ☐ Yes

Describe the exercise:
"On average, how many days per week does patient exercise or do physical activity?" _____

"For how many minutes, on an average day?" _____

b. Smoking

(1) Currently smokes tobacco?

☐ No ☐ Yes

(2) Smoked in past?

☐ No ☐ Yes Year quit: _____

c. Alcohol

(1) How many days per week does patient drink beer, wine or other alcoholic beverages, on average?" _____

(2) If one beer, one glass of wine, or one cocktail equals one drink, how many drinks does patient" have, on an average day?" _____

d. Prescription Medications

☐ No ☐ Yes Please list: _____

_____

_____

_____

e. Non-prescription Medications (check all that apply)

☐ Advil/Aleve
☐ Antacids
☐ Ibuprofen/Naproxen
☐ Anthistamines
☐ Aspirin

☐ Decongestants
☐ Flavonoids
☐ Herbal supplements
☐ Tylenol
☐ Other: _____

_____

_____

Lymphedema Examination continued

PATIENT HISTORY continued

Family History

"(Indicate whether mother, father, brother/sister, aunt/uncle" or grandmother/grandfather and age of onset, if know)"

Heart disease _____

Hypertension _____

Stroke _____

Diabetes _____

Cancer _____

Lymphedema _____

Other _____

Medical tests within the last few years: (check all that apply)

- [ ] ABI
- [ ] Angiogram
- [ ] Arthroscopy
- [ ] Biopsy
- [ ] Blood tests
- [ ] Bone scan
- [ ] Bronchoscopy
- [ ] CT scan
- [ ] Doppler ultrasound
- [ ] Echocardiogram
- [ ] EEG (electrocardiogram)
- [ ] EMG (electromyogram)
- [ ] Lymphscintigraphy
- [ ] Mammogram
- [ ] MRI
- [ ] Myelogram
- [ ] NCV (nerve conduction velocity)
- [ ] Pap smear
- [ ] Pulmonary function test
- [ ] Spinal tap
- [ ] Stool tests
- [ ] "Stress test (eg: treadmill, bicycle)
- [ ] Urine tests
- [ ] X-rays

Past Medical History

Please check if you have ever had:

- [ ] Allergies
- [ ] Arthritis
- [ ] Blood disorders
- [ ] Broken bones/fractures
- [ ] Cancer
- [ ] Circulation problems
- [ ] Depression
- [ ] Developmental/growth problems
- [ ] Diabetes/high blood sugar
- [ ] Head injury
- [ ] Heart problems
- [ ] High blood pressure
- [ ] Infectious disease (ie: tuberculosis, hepatitis)"
- [ ] Kidney problems
- [ ] Low blood sugar/ hypoglycemia
- [ ] Lung problems
- [ ] Multiple sclerosis
- [ ] Muscular dystrophy
- [ ] Osteoporosis
- [ ] Parkinson's disease
- [ ] Repeated infections
- [ ] Seizures/epilepsy
- [ ] Skin diseases
- [ ] Stroke
- [ ] Thyroid problems
- [ ] Ulcers/stomach problems
- [ ] Other:_____

(If history includes cancer, please complete the following)

CANCER TREATMENT PROGRESSION

Include chemotherapy, cancer surgeries, radiation & other interventions"

Date Initiated	Date Completed	Type of Treatment

For Men: Diagonsis of prostate disease?　　[ ] Yes　　[ ] No

For Women: Diagnosis of:

Pelvic inflammatory disease	[ ] Yes	[ ] No
Endometriosis	[ ] Yes	[ ] No
Trouble with menstrual cycle	[ ] Yes	[ ] No
Complicated pregnancies/deliveries	[ ] Yes	[ ] No
Pregnant, or might be pregnant"	[ ] Yes	[ ] No

Current Limitations (check all that apply)

- [ ] Difficulty with locomotion/movement
- [ ] Bed mobility
- [ ] Transfers (ie: moving from bed to chair, bed to toilet, etc.)"
- [ ] Difficulty with self-care (ie: bathing, dressing, toileting)
- [ ] Difficulty with home management (ie: household chores, shopping, driving/transportation)
- [ ] Difficulty sleeping
- [ ] Difficulty with community and work activities/integration
  - [ ] work/school
  - [ ] recreation/play activity
- [ ] Gait
  - [ ] on level
  - [ ] on stairs
  - [ ] on ramps
  - [ ] on uneven terrain

Past Surgery (other than for cancer)　　[ ] Yes　　[ ] No

(If yes, please describe and include dates)

_____　　Month　　Year

_____

_____

Illnesses within the past year: (check all that apply)

- [ ] Bowel problems
- [ ] Chest pains
- [ ] Coordination problems
- [ ] Cough
- [ ] Difficulty sleeping
- [ ] Difficulty swallowing
- [ ] Difficulty walking
- [ ] Dizziness or blackouts
- [ ] Fever/chills/sweats
- [ ] Headaches
- [ ] Hearing problems
- [ ] Heart problems
- [ ] Hoarseness
- [ ] Joint pain or swelling
- [ ] Loss of appetite
- [ ] Loss of balance
- [ ] Nausea/vomiting
- [ ] Pain at night
- [ ] Pain in arms/legs
- [ ] Shortness of breath
- [ ] Urinary problems
- [ ] Vision problems
- [ ] Weakness in arms/legs
- [ ] Weight loss/gain
- [ ] Skin irritation/infection
- [ ] Other: _____
  _____
  _____
  _____

Lymphedema Examination continued

PATIENT HISTORY continued

Current Problems

	Month	Year
When did the problem(s) begin?	☐☐	☐☐☐☐

Describe: _____

_____

_____

Have you ever had the problem(s) before? ☐ Yes ☐ No

If so, what did you do for the problem(s)?_____

_____

Did the problem(s) get better? ☐ Yes ☐ No

About how long did the problem(s) last?_____

How is the problem(s) currently managed?_____

_____

_____

_____

What makes the problem(s) worse? _____

_____

_____

What activities are you not able to do now that you could do before the problem(s)? (Please be as specific as you can; for instance, "Unable to reach over my head".)

_____

_____

_____

_____

_____

_____

What are your goals for treatment? _____

_____

_____

Are you seeing anyone else for the problem(s)? (check all that apply)

☐ Acupuncturist
☐ Cardiologist
☐ Chiropracter
☐ Dentist
☐ Family Practitioner
☐ Internist
☐ Massage Therapist
☐ Neurologist
☐ Nurse
☐ Obstetrician/Gynecologist
☐ Occupational Therapist
☐ Orthopedist
☐ Osteopath
☐ Pediatrician
☐ Physical Therapist
☐ Podiatrist
☐ Primary Care Physician
☐ Rheumatologist

Systems Review

CARDIOVASCULAR—PULMONARY SYSTEM

	Impaired	Not Impaired
	☐	☐

Heart Rate: _____

Blood Pressure: _____

Respiratory Rate: _____

Edema: _____

INTEGUMENTARY SYSTEM Impaired ☐ Not Impaired ☐

Integumentary disruption: _____

Continuity of skin color: _____

Pilability (texture): _____

COMMUNICATION, AFFECT, COGNITION, LEARNING STYLE

	Impaired	Not Impaired
Communication (eg; age-appropriate)	☐	☐
Orientation × 3 (person/place/time)	☐	☐
Emotional/behavior responses	☐	☐

MUSCULOSKELETAL SYSTEM Impaired ☐ Not Impaired ☐

Gross Symmetry:
Standing: _____
Sitting: _____
Activity specific: _____

	Impaired	Not Impaired
Gross Range of Motion:	☐	☐
Gross Strength:	☐	☐

Other: _____

NEUROMUSCULAR SYSTEM Impaired Not Impaired

Gait:

Locomotion: (included transfers, sit-to-stand transitions, bed mobility):	☐	☐

Balance:

Motor function: (motor control, motor learning)	☐	☐

Lymphedema Examination continued

TESTS & MEASUREMENTS

Skin Condition	Yes	No	Comments/Location
Ulcerations			
Contracture			
Dryness			
Other Lesions			
Lipodermatosclerosis			
Hemosiderin			
EDEMA QUALITY			
Pitting			
Non-Pitting			
Fibrotic			
Other:			

Strength/AROM - N/A				
UE	MMT		ROM	
SHOULDER	(R)	(L)	(R)	(L)
Flexion				
Extension				
Abduction				
Adduction				
ER				
IR				
Horiz. AB				
Horiz. AD				
ELBOW				
Flexion				
Extension				
Pronation				
Supination				

Girth (cm)

UE N/A	(R)	(L)	LE N/A	(R)	(L)
MCP			MTP		
Ulnar styloid			Ankle crease		
10cm superior to US			Superior to heel:		
20cm superior to US			10cm		
Olecranon			20cm		
10cm superior to 0			30cm		
20cm superior to 0			40cm		
HAND			Knee joint:		
Thumb: nail bed			Superior to knee joint:		
mid middle phalanx			10cm		
mid prox phalanx			20cm		
Middle finger: nail bed			30cm		
mid middle phalanx			40cm		
mid prox phalanx			50cm		
Ring finger: nail bed			Other:		
mid middle phalanx					
mid prox phalanx					
Small finger: nail bed					
mid middle phalanx					
mid prox phalanx					

Strength/AROM — N/A				
LE	MMT		ROM	
HIP	(R)	(L)	(R)	(L)
Flexion				
Extension				
Abduction				
Adduction				
ER				
IR				
KNEE				
Flexion				
Extension				
ANKLE				
D-flex				
P-flex				
Inv.				
Ev.				

DYNAMOMETER

	(R) 1	2	3	Avg.	(L) 1	2	3
Trial							
Grip strength							
3 jaw chuck							

Sensation:	(R)UE	(L)UE	(R)LE	(L)LE
Intact				
Impaired				
Describe impaired areas:				

POSTURE:

BALANCE:

GAIT:

Reflexes:	N/A
ABI:	N/A

PAIN: Visual Analog Scale:

On the line below, place a mark indicating your pain level:

0 ———————————————————— 10

no pain   worst pain

Lymphedema Examination continued

TESTS & MEASUREMENTS continued

COGNITION & LEARNING PREFERENCES

Understands and can apply basic information:

☐ Yes   ☐ No

Cognitive ability to participate and follow through:

☐ Normal   ☐ Impaired

Learning barriers:

☐ None
☐ Vision
☐ Hearing
☐ Unable to read
☐ Unable to understand what is read
☐ Language/needs interpreter
☐ Other:_____
_____

Education needs:

☐ Disease process   ☐ Skin care
☐ Safety   ☐ Lymphedema bandaging
☐ Use of devices/equipment   ☐ Node clearing
☐ Activities of daily living   ☐ Phase 2 self-management
☐ Exercise program
     Other: _____
_____
_____

How does patient best learn?

☐ Pictures
☐ Reading
☐ Listening
☐ Demonstration
☐ Other: _____
_____
_____

I = Independent with task
A = Assisted task
D = Dependent task
P = Pain

FUNCTIONAL ACTIVITIES ASSESSMENT

I	A	D	P	HYGIENE/GROOMING
				Perform hygiene/grooming tasks
				Commode activities
I	**A**	**D**	**P**	**BATHING**
				Water faucets on/off
				Getting into and out of bath area
				Bathing upper body and/or hair
				Bathing lower body
I	**A**	**D**	**P**	**DRESSING**
				Bend to put on shoes, pants, etc.
				Reach overhead to put on shirt
				Length of time to complete: ( )
				Closures: buttons, zuppers, shoes laces, snaps
				hook & eye, tyoing bow ties, clipping belts
I	**A**	**D**	**P**	**TRANSFERS**
				In & out of bed
				On & off toilet
				On & off chairs, type: ( )
				In & out of car

Lymphedema Examination continued

TESTS & MEASUREMENTS continued

Functional Activities Assessment continued

I = Independent with task
A = Assisted task
D = Dependent task
P = Pain

I	A	D	P	INDEPENDENT LIVING SKILLS
				Reach for items in top cabinet
				Reach for items in low cabinet
				Manipulate pts/pans when cooling
				Carry laundry basket
				Load/unload washer and/or dryer
				Make bed & change linens
				House cleaning (light or heavy)
				Shopping—grocery/mall
				Child care
				Sexual activities
				Yardwork
				Walking: how far? ( )
				Assistive device? What? ( )
				Participate in leisure activities
				Regular exercise
				Adequately pace self during day
				Deal with stress effectively

Community, Home & Work Assessment

Lymphedema Examination

Questionnaire complete: ☐ Yes ☐ No
Photographs taken: ☐ Yes ☐ No
Release form signed: ☐ Yes ☐ No
Patient and/or family in agreement with treatment plan: ☐ Yes ☐ No

EVALUATION

DIAGNOSIS:
(Please mark the appropriate box with #1 for primary, #2 for secondary & #3 for other, as needed)

Musculoskeletal Patterns

☐ A. Primary Prevention/Risk Factor Reduction for Skeletal Demineralization

☐ B. Impaired Posture

☐ C. Impaired Muscle Performance

☐ D. Impaired Joint Mobility, Motor Function, Muscle Performance and Range of Motion Associated with Capsular Restriction

☐ E. Impaired Joint Mobility, Muscle Performance and Range of Motion Associated with Ligament or Other Connective Tissue Disorders

☐ F. Impaired Joint Mobility, Motor Function, Muscle Performance and Range of Motion Associated with Localized Inflammation

☐ G. Impaired Joint Mobility, Motor Function, Muscle Performance and Range of Motion or Reflex Integrity Secondary to Spinal Disorders

☐ H. Impaired Joint Mobility, Muscle Performance and Range of Motion Associated with Fracture

☐ I. Impaired Joint Mobility, Motor Function, Muscle Performance and Range of Motion Associated with Joint Arthroplasty

☐ J. Impaired Joint Mobility, Motor Function, Muscle Performance and Range of Motion Associated with Bony or Soft Tissue Surgical Procedures

☐ K. Impaired Gait, Locomotion, and Balance and Impaired Motor Function Secondary to Lower-Extremity Amputation

Cardiopulmonary Patterns

☐ A. Primary Prevention/Risk Factor Reduction for Cardiopulmonary Disorders

☐ B. Impaired Aerobic Capacity and Endurance Secondary to Deconditioning Associated with Systemic Disorders

☐ C. Impaired Ventilation, Respiration (Gas Exchange), and Aerobic Capacity Associated with Airway Clearance Dysfunction

☐ D. Impaired Aerobic Capacity and Endurance Secondary Cardiovascular Pump Dysfunction

☐ E. Impaired Aerobic Capacity and Endurance Secondary Cardiovascular Pump Failure

☐ F. Impaired Ventilation, Respiration (Gas Exchange), and Aerobic Capacity and Endurance Associated with Ventilatory Pump Dysfunction

☐ G. Impaired Ventilatory with Mechanical Ventilation Secondary to Ventilatory Pump Dysfunction

☐ H. Impaired Ventilation and Respiration (Gas Exhchange) with Potential for Respiratory Failure

☐ I. Impaired Ventilation and Respiration (Gas Exhchange) with Mechanical Ventilation Secondary to Respiratory Failure

☐ J. Impaired Ventilation, Respiration (Gas Exchange), and Aerobic Capacity and Endurance Secondary to Respiratory Failure in the Neonate

Neuromuscular Patterns

☐ A. Impaired Motor Function and Sensory Integrity Associatedwith Congenital or Acquired Disorders of the Central Nervous System in Infancy, Childhood and Adolescence

☐ B. Impaired Motor Function and Sensory Integrity Associated with Acquired Nonprogressive Disorders of the Central Nervous System in Adulthood

☐ C. Impaired Motor Function and Sensory Integrity Associated with Progressive Disorders of the Central Nervous System in Adulthood

☐ D. Impaired Motor Function and Sensory Integrity Associated with Peripheral Nerve Injury

☐ E. Impaired Motor Function and Sensory Integrity Associated with Acute or Chronic Polyneuropathies

☐ F. Impaired Motor Function and Sensory Integrity Associated with Nonprogressive Disorders of the Spinal Cord

☐ G. Impaired Arousal, Range of Motion, Sensory Integrity and Motor Control Associated with Coma, Near Coma or Vegetative State

Integumentary Patterns

☐ A. Primary Prevention/Risk Factor Reduction for Integumentary Disorders

☐ B. Impaired Integumentary Integrity Secondary to Superficial Skin Involvement

☐ C. Impaired Integumentary Integrity Secondary to Partial-Thickness Skin Involvement and Scar Formation

☐ D. Impaired Integumentary Integrity Secondary to Full-Thickness Skin Involvement and Scar Formation

☐ E. Impaired Integumentary Integrity Secondary to kin Involvement Extending into Fascia, Muscle or Bone and Scar Formation

☐ F. Impaired Anthropometric Dimensions Secondary to Lymphatic System Disorders

EVALUATION

PROGNOSIS
(Predicted optimal level of improvement in function, amount of time needed to reach that level.
    If required, these can be referred to as short term and long term goals.)
PLAN OF CARE

Anticipated Goals (_____weeks)

N/A Yes

☐ ☐ Reduce circumferential measurements to within _____ cm of _____ UE/LE
☐ ☐ Improve AROM of _____ UE/LE as follows: _____
☐ ☐ Patient education
☐ ☐ Patient will demonstrate proper skin management
☐ ☐ Patient will demonstrate correct performance of HEP
☐ ☐ Patient will demonstrate adherence to lymphedema precautions
☐ ☐ Reduce pain to _____/10
☐ ☐ Patient will verbalize MLD/CDP program components
☐ ☐ Other:_____

☐ ☐ Other:_____

Expected Outcomes (_____ weeks)

N/A Yes

☐ ☐ Reduce circumferential measurements to within _____ cm of _____ UE/LE
☐ ☐ Improve AROM of _____ UE/LE as follows: _____
☐ ☐ Reduce pain to _____/10
☐ ☐ Patient will demonstrate self-massage techniques
☐ ☐ Postural correction
☐ ☐ Patient will demonstrate independence with self-bandaging with or without assistance
☐ ☐ Patient will demonstrate compression garment donning/doffing/care/wear schedule with or
         without assistance
☐ ☐ Patient voices understanding of need for f/u clinic appointment for assessment of compression
         garment condition/lymphedema status every 4–6 months
☐ ☐ Other: _____
☐ ☐ Other: _____

Frequency of visits/duration of episode of care:

Patient/client to be treated _____ times per week for _____ weeks
    followed by _____

INTERVENTION

Coordination, Communication and Documentation

_____
_____
_____
_____
_____
_____
_____
_____
_____
_____
_____

INTERVENTION continued

Patient/Client Related Instruction

☐ Safety
☐ Exercise
☐ Disease Information

Who was educated?   ☐ Patient   ☐ Family (name and relationship)_____

How did patient/family demonstrate learning:

☐ Patient verbalizes understanding
☐ Family/significant other verbalizes understanding
☐ Patient demonstrates correctly
☐ Demonstration is unsuccessful (describe): _____

_____

_____

DIRECT INTERVENTIONS

	Comments
☐ Manual Lymphatic Drainage	
☐ Lymphedema Bandaging	
☐ HEP/Self-Management Training	
☐ Therapeutic Exercise	
☐ Gait Training	
☐ Education	
☐ Alternative Compression Therapies	
☐ Compression Garment Therapy: Fitting, Evaluation & Alteration	
☐ Other:	
☐ Other:	

Rx		
Performed	**Treatment**	**Comments**
	MLD Region	
	Lymphedema Bandaging	
	HEP/Self-Mgmt. Training	
	Exercise: See protocol	
	Gait Training	
	Education	
	Discussion: Program progression, rationale expectations, bandaging requirements	
	Other:	
	Other:	

Discharge Plan: _____

_____

_____

_____

Signature of therapist _____   **Date** _____

PART II

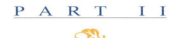

INTERVENTION OPTIONS

Current techniques are surprisingly different from past procedures and are clinically challenging and rewarding for the clinician to deliver. Until the 1980s, patients and health professionals in North America had few options, most of which resulted in a temporary decrease in limb size followed by a return of the signs and symptoms and often worsening of the condition. Patient response has been uniformly positive toward the influx of new knowledge and treatment methods.

Part II of the text will present current intervention options as well as information on education and self-management for the patient with lymphedema. The paradigm shift in intervention will be explained and supported with current literature. Researchers around the world continue to explore and document the fragile yet tenacious nature of the lymphatic system and its response to various interventions.

For some individuals, the use of more than one type of intervention may be indicated. Careful adherence to anatomical and physiological guidelines and attention to confirmed information on human microcirculation may allow selected historical treatment techniques to be delivered with greater success and less compromise to the lymphatic system.

The impact that lymphedema can have on functional ability and quality of life is finally recognized by the medical community. Early diagnosis and accurate intervention can prevent most of the sequelae of this diagnosis. In keeping with the sociomedical model, the health professional must provide the most balanced intervention available, including education and preparation of the patient to assume the self-management portion of the intervention. "Prevention of disability has emerged as a major societal concern for the next century."—Alan Jette[1]

---

[1]Jette, A. M. 1999. Disentangling the process of disablement. *Soc Sci Med.* Feb;48(4):471–72.

4

COMPLETE DECONGESTIVE THERAPY: A FIVE-PART INTERVENTION FOR LYMPHEDEMA

"It was one of the greatest things that has happened to me. It was an instant relief. I thought I was going to have to live with this big arm forever. I learned it can be managed. I felt fortunate to be able to come to the clinic. It was a great experience."

C.S.—PATIENT WITH LYMPHEDEMA FOLLOWING A COURSE OF CDT

"My swelling started one year to the day of surgery. It was painful. With lymphedema therapy, I felt I had regained control of my everyday life. It helped relieve a lot of stress. Treatment taught me how to manage my lymphedema."

K.G.—PATIENT WITH LYMPHEDEMA FOLLOWING A COURSE OF CDT

INTRODUCTION

A treatment program, which came to the forefront in North America in the late 1980s, includes manual techniques as well as lymphedema bandaging to accomplish limb volume reduction and improve connective tissue consistency in the edematous extremity. It is "an effective treatment for lymphedema which results in a normalization of microlymphatic hypertension and an improvement of the clinical appearance."[1] The primary therapeutic advantages that have been proposed include: opening of collateral lymphatic drainage pathways, stimulated pumping by deep lymphatic drainage pathways, and breaking down of excess fibrous tissue.[2,3]

Referred to by several titles, Complete Decongestive Therapy (CDT) (Földi) is a noninvasive treatment, provided by a specially educated health professional. Similar treatments may also be identified as Complex Physical Therapy (Casley-Smith), Combined Decongestive Therapy (Vodder), Complete Decongestive Physiotherapy (CDP), or Combined Physiotherapy (Földi). There is movement in North America toward removing the words *physiotherapy* or *Physical Therapy* from the title since other professionals have entered the treatment arena and may provide similar treatment. A suggestion in 1998 to change the terminology to *Decongestive Lymphatic Therapy (DLT)*[3] has met with mixed reactions in the professional community. CDT is currently the most common designation. This treatment program has been proven safe and effective for over sixty years in Europe and Australia for reducing edematous body parts to normal or near normal size. CDT has been available in North America since the late 1980s but has only recently become well established in most parts of the continent. Evidence for its scientific basis has mounted rapidly in the last ten years, giving the treatment the credibility needed for outcome-based practice models.

A timeline of over one hundred years reflects a strong history of investigation and development of the interventions recommended today:

1890s: Alexander von Winiwarter, a German surgeon, described a treatment for lymphedema that looks much like what is recommended today: conservative treatment that included meticulous cleanliness, compression, massage, and exercise.[4] For a period of time, Winiwarter's treatment suggestions were seemingly forgotten.

1930s: Emil Vodder, PhD, and his wife, Estrid, began working with manual techniques to affect the flow of lymph. Although the Vodders were Danish, the majority of their work was performed and published in France. The term *manual lymph drainage* (MLD) was coined by the Vodders during their years of developing many of the techniques in use today. The Vodder technique of manual lymphatic drainage is the most widely practiced method in North America. It is taught in many of the programs listed in Chapter 8.

1970s: Hungarian physicians, Michael and Ethel Földi, combined Vodder's MLD with lymphedema bandaging, exercise, and specific skin care into what is called Complete Decongestive Physiotherapy (CDP) later rephrased as Complete Decongestive Therapy (CDT). The Földi's work includes extensive research and publications as well as responsibility for directing the Földi Clinic in Germany, which trains German- and English-speaking professionals from around the world.

1980s: First lymphedema treatment center offering CDT opens in North America. Specially educated lymphedema therapists deliver CDT to patients, primarily near large metropolitan areas.

1990s: Proliferation of scientific literature, lymphedema centers, interested physicians, and specially educated lymphedema therapists throughout North America and the world.

2000s: Continued growth in CDT with research focus on quality of life and patient satisfaction issues, cost effectiveness, and controlled clinical studies.

Other medical professionals who have made significant contributions to the field are the late Australian physician John Casley-Smith and his wife, Judith Casley-Smith PhD. The Casley-Smiths have devoted over 40 years to research, education of therapists, and treatment of patients with lymphedema. Their highly regarded research with the electron microscope is prolific and diverse. Albert Leduc, Brussels University, Belgium, has published considerable literature on manual lymph drainage and lymphedema management. His work in isotopic lymphography, in collaboration with his son Oliver Leduc, has established the efficacy of manual techniques in managing lymphedema. There are hundreds of authors whose dedication and quest for answers have led to valuable contributions to the literature. Refer to the individual chapters and the comprehensive reference list at the end of this text for literature by other distinguished contributors.

The information in this chapter should not be used in place of a complete education course in CDT. A high level of competence is needed to adequately deliver the appropriate intervention. The manual techniques require extensive education and practice to master. The lymphedema bandaging techniques require skill to customize and apply correctly. Compression garments are ineffective if not fitted properly. The information needed to deliver these techniques cannot be adequately learned from a book or a videotape alone. Techniques cannot be mastered in a weekend. Individuals interested in learning more about comprehensive education for complete patient intervention should refer to Chapter 8 for a list of education programs.

CDT: TWO-PHASE INTERVENTION FOR LYMPHEDEMA MANAGEMENT

Phase I: Treatment
- Meticulous Skin care
- Manual Lymphatic Drainage
- Lymphedema Bandaging
- Exercise (in bandaging)
- Compression Garment (at the end of Phase I)

Phase II: Self-Management
- Compression Garment (during the day)
- Lymphedema Bandaging (at night)
- Exercise (in garment or bandaging)
- Meticulous Skin care
- Manual Lymphatic Drainage (as needed)

The European model of CDT includes twice daily visits, for an average of 4 to 6 weeks. Due to health care constraints, the North American model is usually limited to daily visits for an average of 3 to 4 weeks to treat a patient with lymphedema of an upper extremity and 4 to 6 weeks to treat a patient with lymphedema of a lower extremity. Some clinics report that due to distances traveled by the patient or numbers of visits limited by payers patients receive CDT three times per week. Despite the limits on visits and other reimbursement issues, professionals involved with the individual with lymphedema should be reminded that reversal of the symptoms is a slow process. Under the best conditions, when appropriate intervention occurs in Phase I and significant patient adherence occurs in Phases I and II, symptom reversal will continue for 18 months or more.[5,6] When rushed or aggressive treatment measures are employed, patients rarely have long-lasting effects and may experience exacerbations of their symptoms due to inappropriate treatment. Individuals with comorbidities may not respond as quickly to treatment due to health problems other than lymphedema.

Meticulous skin care is an essential component of both the treatment phase and the self-management phase. As mentioned in Chapter 2, patients with a limb at risk and those with lymphedema are susceptible to infections through wounds to the skin. The protein-rich fluid that accumulates in the lymphedematous region serves as a bacterial culture for pathogens that are circulating in the body or entering from skin wounds. The goal of such careful attention to the skin is to eliminate or avoid bacterial and fungal growth and subsequent infections such as cellulitis and/or lymphangitis.

Skin care affects the lymph system and the skin by:

- preventing accumulation of bacteria
- assisting in the prevention of secondary infection
- supplying superficial moisture to dry skin
- improving skin suppleness
- reducing hyperkeratosis

References [4,7,8]

Treatment Phase

Patients are taught to be vigilant in inspecting all involved body parts for signs of infection or inflammation as well as skin wounds. A list of precautions should be provided early on in the treatment phase to help the patient avoid compromising situations. An example of a handout, which can be provided for the patient, is included in Chapter 8. Cleansing, moisturizing, and protection techniques are taught and practiced during the treatment phase. Involved skin is covered with an appropriate moisturizer before lymphedema bandaging is applied.

Self-Management Phase

Patients assume responsibility for managing and maintaining skin health during this phase. Patient adherence to a daily regime of appropriate cleansing and moisturizing of the involved areas will assist in the prevention of infection over his or her lifetime.

Manual Lymph Drainage (MLD) is an approach based on the physiologic principles of lymph flow and lymph vessel emptying. Manual techniques include ipsilateral and contralateral treatment in lymph node regions to facilitate lymph flow into adjacent body areas. The use of lymphography and lymphscintigraphy for research and diagnostic purposes has confirmed that superficially lymph fluid will move opposite to natural flow patterns, around blocked areas and into more central vessels with the use of these specialized manual techniques. MLD addresses primarily the superficial or initial lymphatics to influence lymph circulation. MLD affects the lymph system by:

- increasing the frequency of lymph vessel contractions through mild stimulation
- increasing the volume of lymph fluid that is transported
- increasing pressure in the lymph collector vessels
- improving lymph transport capacity
- reversing the direction of flow from natural flow patterns toward collateral vessels, anastomoses, and uninvolved lymph node regions
- increasing arterial blood flow. This, under investigation now, may prove to enhance angiogenesis and thereby increase the number of available, functioning lymphatics

References [1,2,5,9–14]

Treatment Phase

Treatment is delivered to the patient in a recumbant position whenever possible for comfort and to further facilitate lymph fluid movement. MLD will engage the use of functioning lymph nodes and vessels adjacent to the regions that are not functioning adequately. Consequently, regardless of the site of lymph system damage, treatment includes manual work on the neck, back, abdominal region, and uninvolved inguinal and axillary lymph nodes, initially moving from the contralateral trunk area toward the congested area. Finally, treatment moves from the involved area toward the uninvolved areas. All clothing is removed and the patient is draped for privacy and warmth. If the patient cannot achieve prone positioning for treatment of the back, cannot tolerate supine positioning, or is unable to roll, the treatment can be delivered in a modified position. The manual techniques delivered by MLD are light and specific, requiring specialized education to be delivered accurately. They are *not* the strokes and pressures used in *effluerage,* a standard massage technique used in therapeutic massage treatments. The MLD portion of the treatment session will usually require a minimum of 30 to 60 minutes, depending on the size of the limb(s), the severity of the symptoms, and the amount of fibrosis.

Self-Management Phase

Patients are taught some manual techniques as appropriate, to assist in self-management of the condition. Excessive pressure can cause exacerbation of symptoms; therefore, patients who appear able to participate in the manual therapy must be screened and instructed carefully. If a patient experiences an increase in swelling or a plateau in reduction following the treatment phase, it is appropriate to follow up with additional sessions of MLD in the clinic. At this point, manual therapy may further enhance the gains achieved during the initial treatment phase. The patient returning with increased swelling should be examined and cleared for possible malignancy or other complications before continuing treatment.

FIGURE 4-1 Demonstration of Manual Lymph Drainage Technique

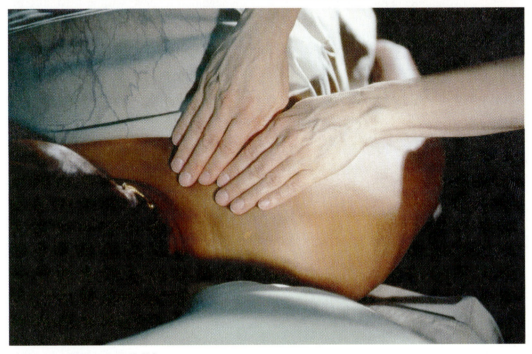

(Courtesy of Deborah G. Kelly)

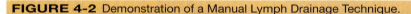

FIGURE 4-2 Demonstration of a Manual Lymph Drainage Technique.

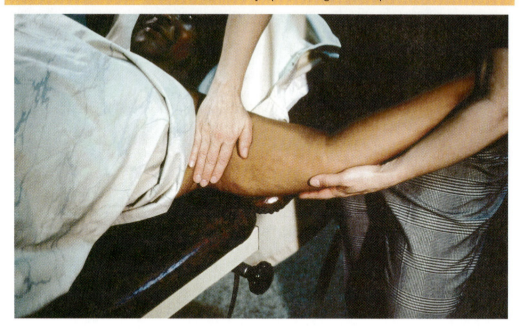

(Courtesy of Deborah G. Kelly)

Lymphedema bandaging is credited by management experts with at least 50% of the success of the treatment phase. Elasticity of the cutaneous tissues is partially lost in lymphedema. Tissue hydrostatic pressures must be maintained by the use of external support. This support must be continuous until the tissues can regain their elasticity and assume their role in maintaining tissue pressures. During the treatment phase, the support is best provided by specialized bandaging. A specific combination of short-stretch bandages, padding, and foam are applied in layers following each session of MLD. The bandaging techniques affect the lymphatic system because they:

- provide a mild increase in tissue pressure, which assists lymph vessels to empty
- prevent refilling of the interstitium with fluid between treatments by reducing the hydrostatic pressure gradient from blood to the tissues
- provide support for tissues that have lost elasticity
- facilitate colloidal protein reabsorption
- reduce the rate of ultrafiltration
- improve the efficiency of the muscle pump during muscle activity
- provide localized pressure when indicated to soften fibrotic tissue

References [1,9,15–20]

Treatment Phase

It is important to distinguish between short-stretch (or low-elastic) bandages and long-stretch (or high-elastic) bandages and the type of compression that each offers.[21] For more information on where to obtain short-stretch bandages see Chapter 8.

Short-stretch Bandages	Long-stretch Bandages
Form a strong support during muscle contraction. Total tissue pressure is significantly raised.	Due to their extensibility, do not provide much resistance during muscle contraction. Total tissue pressure is not significantly raised during muscle contraction.
Do not constrict during rest.	Long-stretch bandages such as Ace® bandages provide a high resting pressure, which is contraindicated based on lymph vessel physiology and function. When applied firmly, they may provide an uncomfortable level of constriction during rest.

Though the bandages are bulky, patients can and should maintain if not increase their activity level while wearing them to facilitate muscle pumping and general function. After a period of adjustment, most motivated patients tolerate the bandages well. For optimum patient adherence, patients should be thoroughly educated about the importance of the lymphedema bandaging portion of the treatment phase. Most patients report that the cosmetic appearance of the bandaging is more challenging to overcome than mobility or comfort issues. The bandages are worn 23 hours a day during the treatment phase. Patients and their families learn how to apply their own bandages toward the middle of the treatment phase.

The bandaging portion of the treatment session may take a minimum of 15 to 90 minutes depending on the number of custom foam pieces that are needed, how much patient education is indicated, how many limbs are affected, the size of the involved limb(s), how many skin lesions require care, and how much assistance is required for bandaging. By the second or third week of the treatment phase, the amount of clinician time spent bandaging should be reduced but may still require alterations in custom pieces, patient education, and changes in application due to patient progress.

Specialized education is required to accurately and safely apply the lymphedema bandaging. Patients should be regularly monitored by a qualified health care professional. With the correct application, the bandaging is safe and effective. If the bandages are applied incorrectly, complications may arise.

Self-Management Phase

Patients learn how to use the bandaging techniques to manage their condition once the treatment phase has ended. The severity and chronicity of the symptoms will determine whether a patient should continue to wear the bandaging at night after the treatment phase has ended. Most individuals apply the bandaging at night to optimize reductions during the self-management phase. Patients report that their symptoms can fluctuate with changes in lifestyle, climate, and body weight. Most agree that their condition is best controlled with consistent use of all components of the self-management phase but that occasional lapses in adherence can be addressed by following their home program more closely.

Exercises are performed in Phase I while wearing the lymphedema bandaging. Later, these exercises are performed in a compression garment during the

FIGURE 4-3 Example of Lymphedema Bandaging for the Upper Extremity

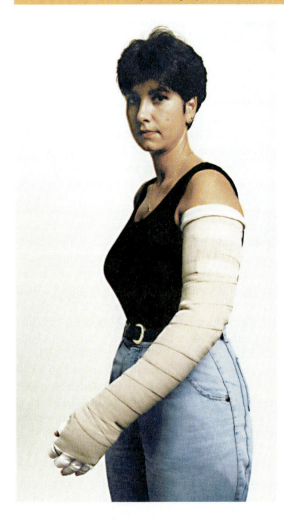

(Courtesy of Lohmann & Rauscher, Inc.)

self-management phase. The exercise program will include activities that promote emptying of lymph regions, which are centrally located and adjacent to the involved regions, as well as activities to assist the remaining lymphatics to work more effectively. Exercise affects the lymph system by:

- increasing lymph vessel contractions
- improving the circulation of lymph fluid through body movement
- enhancing the efficiency of fluid transport by the thoracic duct through deep breathing
- varying total tissue pressures via muscle contractions
- assisting in maintenance of normal tissue hydrostatic pressure
- preventing further accumulation of fluid

References [7,9,15,22,23,24]

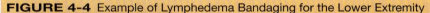

FIGURE 4-4 Example of Lymphedema Bandaging for the Lower Extremity

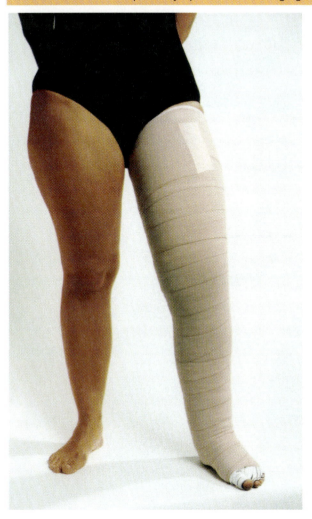

(Courtesy of Lohmann &
Rauscher, Inc.)

Treatment Phase

The goal of exercise is twofold: to improve or support lymphatic function and to improve or support the patient's level of ability. Patients are instructed in an exercise program that is customized to their level of functional ability. The exercise program should take into account limitations uncovered during the examination process. Due to the disabling nature of carrying one or more enlarged limbs, most patients with lymphedema experience some level of limitation in joint range of motion, muscle strength, and posture. When lymphedema is triggered by failure of another body system (such as venous insufficiency), that system will also be addressed with exercise during the treatment phase. Any limitations found during the examination should be addressed in the exercise program. To assist the patient in carrying out the exercise program

FIGURE 4-5 Patient Performing Self-bandaging Techniques to the Lower Extremity

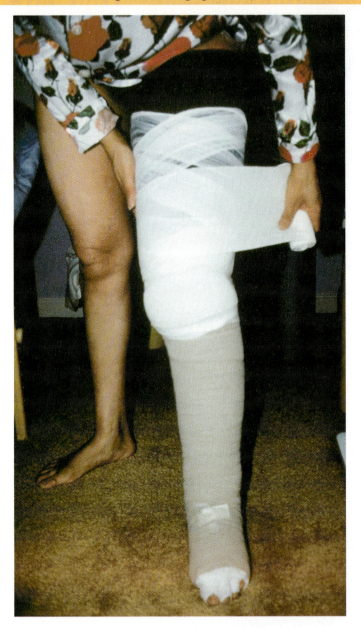

(Courtesy of Deborah G. Kelly)

during the self-management phase, an on-site video can be made of the patient performing the exercises during the treatment phase. Videos with general exercise programs for upper- and lower-extremity lymphedema can also be purchased by the patient. See Chapter 8.

FIGURE 4-6 Instructor Applying Lymphedema Bandaging to the Lower Extremity of a Patient Volunteer during a Classroom Demonstration

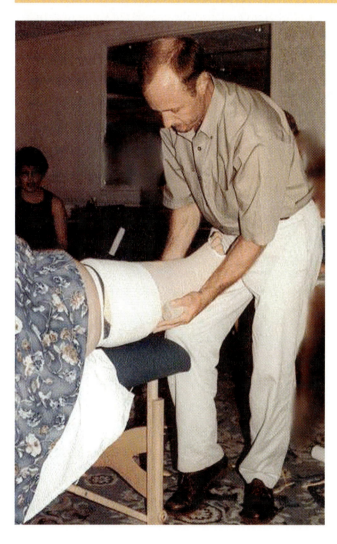

(Courtesy of Klose Norton Training & Consulting, LLC)

The amount of time spent on exercise during a session in the treatment phase will vary, based on the number of limitations measured and the intervention goals. If there are no other existing functional limitations, a patient may be able to take over the primary responsibility for exercise even during the treatment phase.

In addition to prescribed exercise, incorporating recreational exercise into weekly activities is also important for weight control and cardiac fitness. Patients are encouraged to participate in carefully selected activities outside of therapy sessions. Investigation into the benefits of exercise to manage fatigue following cancer treatment have shown that aerobic exercise can be beneficial.[25,26] Some activities have been shown to increase the likelihood of developing lymphedema or worsening the condition.[27] Examples reported by patients include golf, tennis, cross country skiing, and ambitious weight lifting. The topic of exercise is currently controversial among health care professionals. Participation in recreational activities can enhance overall fitness levels and improve quality of life perceptions. Because of the value of activity, some health professionals are reluctant to caution patients about limiting activities without extensive scientific evidence to support them. Until more data is collected, patients should be presented with current information and assisted in making decisions about what activities will be most beneficial for them. To educate patients on how to assess exercise options, they should be advised to *avoid activities that can trigger a further decrease of the transport capacity of the lymph vessels and/or unnecessarily increase the lymphatic fluid and protein load of the lymphatic system in the affected region.*[28]

During vigorous, repetitive exercise, it is normal for local hyperemia to occur, leading to alterations in local metabolism. Performing *unaccustomed eccentric* exercise will result in a number of physiological responses, including delayed onset muscle soreness (*DOMS*). Although the specific cause is not known, *DOMS* does appear to be linked to eccentric muscle activation. For the person with a normal lymphatic system, the presence of muscle soreness alone is not an indication that the exercise should be discontinued. After the initial insult to unaccustomed activity, a tolerance factor emerges.[29] For the person with lymphedema or a limb at risk, however, *DOMS* may be viewed as a reminder that local metabolism is being altered. It would be prudent to minimize the opportunity for *DOMS* to occur in an exercise session for the individual with lymphedema or a limb at risk. The exercise program should concentrate on smooth, rhythmic, *concentric* activities with light resistance. Swimming is an ideal exercise choice because there is minimal *eccentric* behavior during this activity. Other benefits of swimming, related to the hydrostatic pressure of water, have been discussed in previous chapters.

In the individual with a normal lymphatic system, excess metabolites and water are removed efficiently following exercise. For the individual with an impaired lymphatic system, exercise programs that increase the likelihood of localized hyperemia may trigger the onset or the exacerbation of symptoms. Since there is currently no efficient method of predicting who will develop lymphedema, everyone at risk, sedentary or physically fit, should be educated about the risks. Exercise programs should be compatible with the fitness level of the patient, while serving to enhance circulation of lymph fluid.

Some of the variables that would affect the decision about the type, frequency, and intensity of exercise are:

- **Age**—The older the individual, the more predisposed they will be to cardiovascular disorders, poor peripheral blood distribution, orthostatic hypotension, decreased aerobic capacity, and decreased overall exercise capacity.[30]
- **Overall level of health and fitness**—The more sedentary the individual, the higher the degree of DOMS and other responses to the introduction of exercise.
- **Side of lymph vessel involvement versus side of body that the activity would stress**—A right-handed tennis serve may not stress the left axillary area.
- **Level of skill in the activity in question**—Is this a new exercise or one that the individual has been performing regularly for some time?

- **Level of intensity that the activity requires**—The higher the intensity, the greater the local hyperemic response to exercise.
- **Is the exercise more eccentric** (lengthening against resistance) **or concentric** (shortening against a load)?—A muscle produces the least force when contracting concentrically.
- **Location of radiation treatment if applicable**—Irradiated tissues are not as extensible.

Instruction in achieving a balance between exercise and rest as well as overall energy conservation strategies should be included in all exercise programs. A recent study maintains that women who have undergone axillary dissection and radiation for the treatment of breast cancer *may* be able to safely participate in strenuous activity.[31] It was unclear, however, if the subjects in this study were physically fit before initiating the exercise regime or if the exercise activity was one they had previously performed. Long-term follow-up was not available to report possible onset or exacerbation of symptoms after the study. Clinicians should assist in making exercise decisions based on the criteria given until further studies have followed subjects of all types and fitness levels for an extended period of time. Health professionals knowledgeable about the complexities of exercise should be included in the intervention plan for an individual with lymphedema.

Self-Management Phase

Patients are encouraged to continue with their exercise program during the self-management phase. Exercise is usually performed in the compression garment during this phase. Periodic clinic visits may be needed to revise the home program or adjust for improvements or decline in function. The goal of the exercise program should be to maximize both functional ability and the circulation of lymph fluid.

Compression garments are fitted at the end of the treatment phase when the involved limb(s) have reached normal or near normal size. The elastic support garments are worn during the day to prevent the re-accumulation of fluid. The application of a compression garment affects the lymph system by:

- providing long-term preservation of reduced limb circumferences
- preventing refilling of interstitium with fluid by contributing to hydrostatic pressure control
- providing extracellular tissue pressures to facilitate fluid uptake and continued softening of fibrotic tissues initiated during the treatment phase
- providing support for tissues that have lost elasticity due to the disease process

References [4,18,32]

Treatment Phase

A compression garment is appropriate for the patient at the end of the treatment phase. A specially educated individual with a full understanding of the disease process is most qualified to make the detailed decisions about garment selection. Specific education is needed to determine the correct garment style, appropriate pressure gradient, and fit for each person's needs. Without involvement of the educated individual, much

FIGURE 4-7 Patient Performing Lower Extremity Exercise with a Ball While Wearing Lymphedema Bandaging

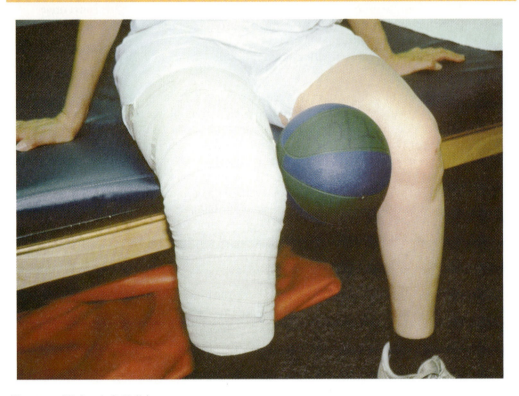

(Courtesy of Deborah G. Kelly)

time and money can be wasted in attempts to provide a patient with an appropriate garment. Many patients report poor results while using a compression garment simply because the fit and application were performed incorrectly. (See Chapter 8 for list of contacts for garments.)

Because they are highly elastic, compression garments allow for some swelling of the tissues and are not recommended for nightwear unless the patient is unable to tolerate the lymphedema bandaging at night. The compression garment application enters the treatment plan near the end of this phase but is, nonetheless, a part of the treatment. There is evidence that without the use of the compression garment, treatment results from Phase I and long-term results from Phase II will be significantly limited. *Without adequate patient education and adherence, proper fitting techniques, and effective monitoring, the compression garment will not be an effective part of the treatment.*

Self-Management Phase

During the self-management phase, the patient will wear the compression garment during daytime hours, changing to lymphedema bandaging for night time. By the end of the treatment phase, the patient should know donning, doffing, and garment care information. Patients should also remain alert to any changes in the tissue adjacent to the garment edges. Tissue swelling and fibrosis can occur in nearby areas if garments

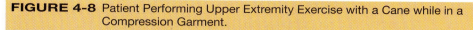

FIGURE 4-8 Patient Performing Upper Extremity Exercise with a Cane while in a Compression Garment.

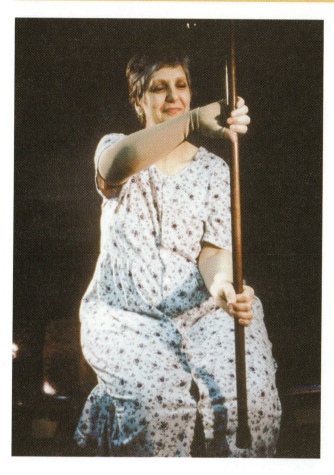

(Courtesy of Deborah G. Kelly)

do not fit well. Patients may be taught lymph node clearing techniques to use along with the garment to enhance lymph vessel function and prevent complications. Many patients will need to wear a compression garment for the remainder of their lives to effectively control symptoms and retain their limb reduction. Garment fit and condition should be checked every 6 months or sooner if the patient experiences difficulties with fit, comfort level, or control of the symptoms.

Compression garment summary:

- Avoid use of garment until the end of the treatment phase when optimal or near-normal limb reduction has been reached.
- Recognize the use of the garment as essential for long-term management of swelling caused by lymphedema and educate patients about this information.
- Select a specially educated professional to measure, select the compression grade, and fit garments.

FIGURE 4-9 Example of a Medical Compression Garment: Jobst Elvarex® Upper Extremity Medical Compression Garment

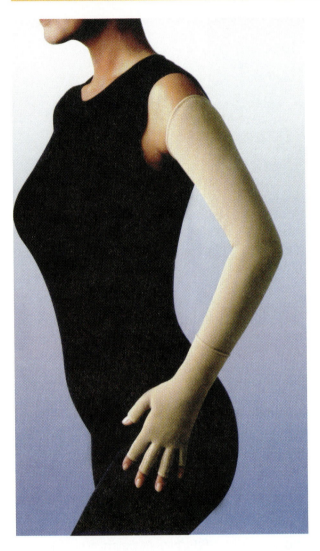

(Courtesy of BSN-Jobst Inc.)

- Use garments specifically designed for management of lymphedema. (The fabric, pressure gradient, style, and quality should all be geared toward the unique needs of the individual with lymphedema.)
- Replace every 6 months or sooner if garment is stretched.
- Consider wearing prophylactically during air travel and other periods of prolonged immobility or pressure change. This may be especially important for the person with subclinical evidence of lymphedema but no measurable swelling.
- Wash regularly. Have a second set to alternate washing and wearing cycles.

FIGURE 4-10 Pediatric Patient Wearing Medical Compression Garments

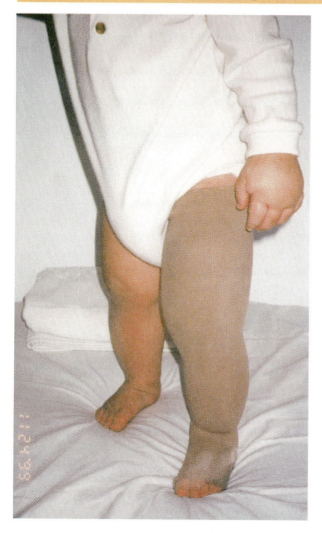

(Courtesy of Klose Norton Training & Consulting, LLC)

- Consider selecting a lower pressure gradient for a garment, in some cases, to improve patient adherence. A garment in the drawer is not doing its job. Someone who has a difficult time applying a snug garment may be less likely to continue to wear it.

The principles of lymph flow, lymph load, and volume apply to all types of swelling whether they are acute, chronic, or permanent conditions. The five-part treatment program and the self-management techniques introduced here can be used in part or total for patients with other types of edema and a variety of diagnoses. Special precautions not listed in this text must be considered when applying CDT to diagnoses other than lymphedema. Consult a specifically educated lymphedema therapist for more information.

Indications for CDT include but are not limited to:

- Lymphedema
- Lipedema (Bilateral, symmetrical swelling, primarily of the lower extremities[33])
- Chronic Venous Insufficiency
- Post-thrombotic conditions
- CRPS—Complex Regional Pain Syndrome (Formerly known as RSD—Reflex Sympathetic Dystrophy)
- Traumatic Edema (Iatrogenic, post-surgical, post-musculoskeletal injury)
- Rheumatoid Arthritis (RA)
- Chronic wounds

Complete decongestive therapy is compatible with anatomical and physiological principles. The majority of patients with lymphedema experience satisfying results with this type of intervention. If patients are adherent to the program during both phases, they may continue to have reductions in limb volume and improvement in connective tissue quality for at least two years after Phase I has ended. Those who do not progress may fall into one of the following categories:

Lack of progress—Phase I: Treatment Phase

- Patient has malignant lymphedema. CDT may be indicated as palliative care but results will be less dramatic.
- Significant amounts of fibrotic tissue can slow treatment progression. Changes may be noted over months or years instead of days or weeks.
- Self-induced lymphedema. For more information on this topic refer to Weissleder.[22]
- Treatment applied was insufficient—that is, bandaging applied improperly, MLD used but not bandaging, bandaging applied but no MLD used, MLD too aggressive.
- Patient presents with associated illness that complicates reversal of symptoms, such as obesity or lipedema.
- Patient does not adhere to the program during treatment phase.
- Patient is using pneumatic compression pump without observing precautions for use as listed in Chapter 5.
- Patient has cognitive impairments associated with a secondary illness, which limit adherence with the treatment.
- Therapist is unskilled or newly skilled in CDT techniques.

Lack of progress—Phase II: Self-management Phase

- Patient does not adhere to the prescribed program during the self-management phase.
- There is a recurrence of cancer.

- Patient presents with new or recurrent illness.
- Patient is using pneumatic compression pump without observing precautions for use as listed in Chapter 5.
- As previously noted, significant amounts of fibrotic tissue can slow treatment progression. Changes may be noted over months or years instead of days or weeks.
- Genital, head, and neck edemas tend to have less satisfying results with rapid return of swelling unless the patient adheres diligently to the prescribed program during this phase.

Precautions and contraindications to CDT treatments should be discussed with the patient and referring physician. Inform the referring physician that the treatment will cause a *temporary increase in circulating blood volume.* For most patients with the diagnoses below, the treatment will still be indicated but with close monitoring of cardiac and pulmonary functions.

I. **Precautions and relative contraindications:**
    A. Acute infections—Local or systemic, viral or bacterial: cellulitis, erysipelas, other secondary acute inflammation.
    B. Uncontrolled bronchial asthma.
    C. Cardiac edema—Work with referring physician, consider an EKG for more information.
    D. Malignancy—Work with the oncologist and the patient to make treatment decisions.
    E. Acute bronchitis—Wait until the symptoms have decreased.
    F. If the patient has had cancer treatment in the past, and symptoms of lymphedema worsen during the treatment phase or patient's health declines, refer to oncologist and suspect recurrence of cancer.
    G. Renal insufficiency.
    H. Hypertension.

II. **MLD contraindications:**
    A. **Neck** treatment
        1. Cardiac arrhythmia—Can create arrhythmia by stimulating receptors.
        2. Patients over age 60—Arteries and veins often become sclerotic with age.
        3. Hyperthyroidism or hypothyroidism.
        4. Hypersensitivity of the carotid sinus.
    B. **Abdominal** treatment
        1. Pregnancy.
        2. Menstrual period (relative).
        3. Abdominal surgery (recent)—Check with physician.
        4. Complications to the abdominal area or its contents following radiation therapy—Chronic inflammation, fibrosis.
        5. Crohn's disease, diverticulitis, or undiagnosed abdominal pain of any kind.

6. Aortic aneurysm or suspicious symptoms such as complaints of low back pain or palpation of a strong aortic pulse.
7. Diabetes—Be cautious, some blood vessels become sclerotic during the disease process.

C. **Lower extremity** treatment
1. Deep vein thrombosis—Conservative management usually allows six months resolution of symptoms before beginning MLD. *Physicians more knowledgeable about CDT now support the use of MLD as early as two weeks after the initial thrombus.* Work closely with referring practitioner to establish approval of early intervention. Expect a slower response to treatment; avoid deep strokes.
2. Phlebitis or thrombophlebitis.

Clinical Implications: No scientific study has ever shown that the application of manual techniques accelerates the spread of cancer cells or the growth of tumors. Since many cancer treatments target cells in the general circulation, any treatment that improves circulation of lymph or blood will usually be recommended, not avoided.

III. Lymphedema bandaging precautions
A. Lower extremity arterial disease—Work closely with referring practitioner; if indicated, seek calculation of the ABI. Compression is contraindicated at an ABI of <0.8. See Chapter 3 for a description of this noninvasive assessment of lower extremity circulation.
B. Acute infection such as cellulitis.
C. Use caution and work with physician if diagnoses include:
1. hypertension
2. paralysis
3. diabetes
4. asthma
5. malignant lymphedema
6. cor pulmonale—right-sided heart failure and left-sided heart failure with pulmonary edema. (The general term *congestive heart failure* (CHF) is used but is less accurate and descriptive.)

SUMMARY

CDT has been successful for over 60 years in safely and effectively treating the signs and symptoms of lymphedema. There is adequate scientific literature as well as empirical and anecdotal evidence for the efficacy of the intervention. Specific education is required to master the skills needed to deliver adequate intervention. A major component of CDT is education and preparation for the self-management phase. Investigation is still needed to support and compare cost, efficacy, adherence, satisfaction, and quality of life associated with different intervention strategies.

CASE 4–1 PRIMARY LYMPHEDEMA (TARDA), STAGE III, LYMPHOSTATIC ELEPHANTIASIS

PD is a patient with an extraordinary case of primary lymphedema of the left lower extremity. In 1996, PD, age 56, presented to a treatment clinic in Princeton, New Jersey, with lymphostatic elephantiasis, or Stage III lymphedema. She had no other serious health concerns at this time and had well-controlled diabetes. She had no family history of lymphedema.

PD emigrated from Jamaica to the United States in 1979. In 1980, she began to notice a persistent but mild swelling in the left foot and ankle. The leg progressively swelled without any apparent cause and without a suitable diagnosis until 1996.

Remarkably, until this time, the affected leg was not treated with any of the so-called "standard treatments" such as diuretics, compression gradient stockings, pneumatic compression pumps, or surgeries. The patient reported that the physicians with whom she consulted were so uncertain as to the nature of the condition that they remained reluctant to employ any treatment measures. As the leg became more massively swollen, a debulking surgery was recommended, but the patient was uncomfortable with this plan of action.

Before 1994, PD reported no incidence of infection in the affected areas. Beginning in 1994, and at a point where the lymphedema had progressed to Stage III, PD suffered her first episode of cellulitis. In the next two years she was hospitalized six times for 3 to 4 weeks duration each time, and felt as though she was "constantly fighting an infection." With the use of antibiotics and having become familiar with the early signs and symptoms of cellulitis, PD was able to self-administer the necessary medicines, as required. This allowed the severity of each bout to be greatly limited. PD reports that she still required nearly continual antibiotic support.

Even with a massively swollen leg, she continued in her employment as a nurse's aide in a senior citizens home. As the frequency of infections increased, she was forced into a nearly continual, nonambulatory status, discontinued her employment, and was put on permanent disability. Following each infectious episode, the patient's symptoms of lymphedema were severely and irreversibly worsened. Several biopsies were performed but results were inconclusive. One physician recommended amputation at this time.

In November 1996, a parasitologist recommended CDT. At the start of treatment the patient's weight was 305+ pounds; however, she did not appear to be obese. She presented with multiple lobular outgrowths on the medial and posterior thigh and posterior calf, and tremendous overall limb girth. The foot was minimally involved. The circumferential measurements of her leg at the largest point of the thigh were more than 135.5 cm (see chart). The right leg exhibited no signs of lymphedema with no adipose tissue.

Treatment was administered 2×/day, 5 days/week. The intensive phase, without interruption, was of seven months' duration and consisted of more than 250 treatment sessions. At the end of this intensive phase, the patient's treatment schedule was modified to 1×/day, and later to 3–4× per week. The patient was instructed to remain continuously compressed in multilayered, short-stretch cotton bandaging materials during the second phase (homecare optimization phase) due to the loss of tissue pressure within the decongested limb.

It had been noted that any inconsistency in compression resulted in rapid refilling of the affected areas. The circumference following the intensive phase was decreased by 70+ cm at the most affected point. Overall weight loss was 96 pounds. It was also noted during the course of treatment that the previously unaffected leg began to exhibit mild swelling. The patient was fitted with a compression stocking for the previously unaffected leg and treatment guidelines were modified to rely less on the contralateral inguinal lymph nodes.

During the homecare phase, PD was instructed to rewrap her leg after showering, and to remain in compression bandaging continuously. After 3 to 4 months it was noted that tissue stabilization was occurring. She was then fitted with a gradient compression stocking. As a safeguard she was instructed to wear this garment with caution and for short periods of time only. The patient noticed that some refilling would occur within the stocking and opted to wear it on special occasions only.

At this time a plastic surgeon, who had an appreciation for the complexities and the pathology of lymphedema, was consulted. PD's former lobular outgrowths were now decongested and, as expected, much shrinkage in the flaccid skin areas was noted. Further spontaneous reduction in these skin areas was not expected and the patient desired a cosmetic improvement. In October 1997 the first of four skin excision surgeries was performed. The surgical approach was timed to coincide with a thoroughly decongested skin area, and

was performed in the least aggressive fashion involving relatively small "target" areas. All incisions were performed longitudinally and parallel to the existing lymphatic vessels. A second surgery occurred in December of 1997, a third in February of 1998, and the fourth in August of 1998. The staging of these procedures was deemed necessary to prevent blood loss and promote more complete and thorough healing of the incision site.

At present, due to lack of insurance reimbursement, PD receives only periodic CDT treatments. She manages her lymphedema as would most patients in the following fashion: daily donning of her medical compression stocking, nightly doffing of the garment, followed by self-administered compression bandaging of the entire leg from toe to groin. MLD is not performed by the patient and no congestion is noted within the leg; however, there is a chronic enlargement beyond normal due to the retention of lymphostatic fibrosis. The patient is very satisfied with the intervention outcomes. She has not suffered an infectious episode since she began CDT treatment in November 1996. See Figures 4.11 a–d.

Measurement Chart: PD

Date:	11/25/96	11/25/96	5/9/00	5/9/00	
Distance from Heel:	**Right Leg**	**Left Leg**	**Right Leg**	**Left Leg**	**Reduction**
79	58.7	133	65.8	73.4	59.6
62	52.4	135.5	53.2	72.3	63.2
47	37.8	77.6	39.9	50	27.6
32	34.5	84.4	38.6	45	39.4
19	28	71.8	29.8	35	36.8
9	23.2	33.6	24.4	23.4	10.2
Dorsm	22.5	28.8	22.3	24.5	43.3
Weight:	305+ lb.		209 lb.		96 lb.

Submitted by Günter Klose, certified instructor, MLD/CDT and Steve Norton, instructor, MLD/CDT, cofounders of Klose Norton Training and Consulting, LLC.

FIGURE 4-11a Primary Lymphedema, Left Lower Extremity, Before Intervention

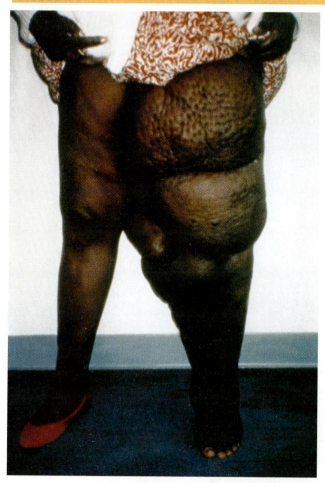

(Courtesy of Klose Norton Training & Consulting, LLC)

FIGURE 4-11b Primary Lymphedema, Left Lower Extremity, Before Intervention

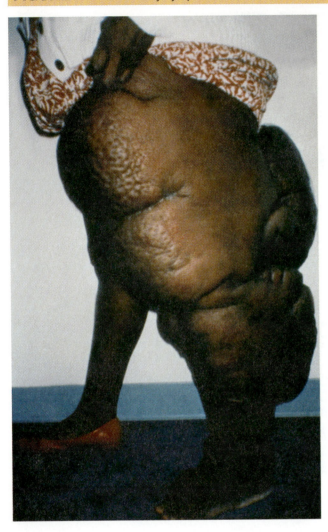

(Courtesy of Klose Norton Training & Consulting, LLC)

FIGURE 4-11c Primary Lymphedema, Left Lower Extremity, after Complete Decongestive Therapy (CDT)

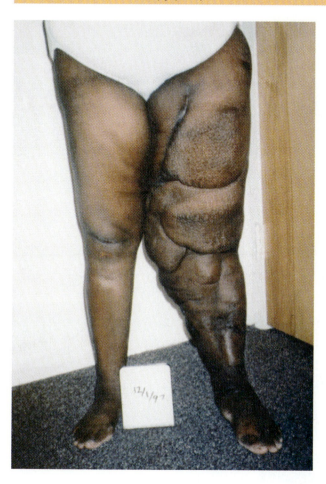

(Courtesy of Klose Norton Training & Consulting, LLC)

FIGURE 4-11d Primary Lymphedema, Left Lower Extremity, after Complete Decongestive Therapy (CDT)

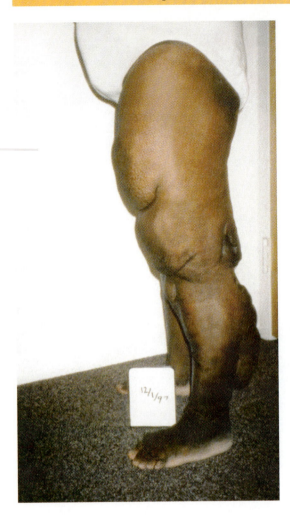

(Courtesy of Klose Norton Training & Consulting, LLC)

CASE 4–2 SECONDARY LYMPHEDEMA, BILATERAL LOWER EXTREMITIES

EH is a 50-year-old male with IDDM, s/p Right BKA, May 1999. The patient suffered recurrent infections (cellulitis) since 1993 in both lower extremities. Patient developed lymphedema secondary to chronic infection. Symptoms of lymphedema were exacerbated with each episode of infection and were significantly worse by September 1999. Right stump swelling continued to increase until incision *dehisced* (burst open) during a prosthesis fitting session with a prosthetist. The resulting wound on the posterior portion of the stump measured 2 cm by 2.5 cm. CDT was initiated in October 1999. A total of twenty-two treatments were performed. Wound care was included in the five-part intervention. Wound dressings included antibiotic ointment, adaptic gauze, 4×4s, and Kerlix. To maintain the limb reductions achieved with CDT, the patient was fitted with a Juzo® stump shrinker, compression Class 2 (30–40 mm Hg) for the right lower extremity, and a thigh-high stocking compression Class 2 for the left lower extremity. By December 1999, the patient was fitted with a new prosthesis to be applied over the stump shrinker. The prosthetist attended several of the CDT sessions to better understand the intervention process and to learn how to best accommodate for the patient's special needs.

Measurements in centimeters

	Left lower extremity		Right lower extremity	
	10/18/99	11/16/99	10/18/99	11/16/99
MT base	24.5	24.3		
4 cm above	25.7	24.5		
8 cm above	29.0	26.7		
Malleoli	31.5	29.0		
4 cm above	32.0	25.8		
8 cm above	36.0	27.5		
12 cm	38.8	30.5		
16 cm	43.0	34.0	26.5	21.0
20 cm	46.8	38.0	38.0	31.5
24 cm	48.5	39.3	43.5	35.8
28 cm	46.5	39.0	44.0	36.8
32 cm	44.5	38.4	42.9	38.5
36 cm	43.5	39.3	44.8	40.8
40 cm	47.3	43.1	47.0	44.8
44 cm	50.5	44.5	47.7	44.8
48 cm	52.5	46.5	51.8	46.0
52 cm	55.5	50.0	55.3	49.0
56 cm	58.0	53.5	57.0	53.0

See Figures 4.12 a–c.

Submitted by Barbara Ann DeOlden-Murphy, MSPT, MLD/CDT and Carrie Sullivan, PTA, MLD/CDT. Guthrie Lymphedema Clinic, Guthrie Healthcare Systems, Sayre, Pennsylvania.

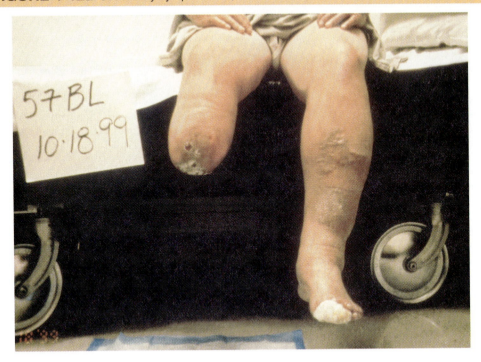

(Courtesy of Guthrie Healthcare System: Guthrie Lymphedema Clinic)

FIGURE 4-12b Secondary Lymphedema, Bilateral Lower Extremities, after Complete Decongestive Therapy (CDT)

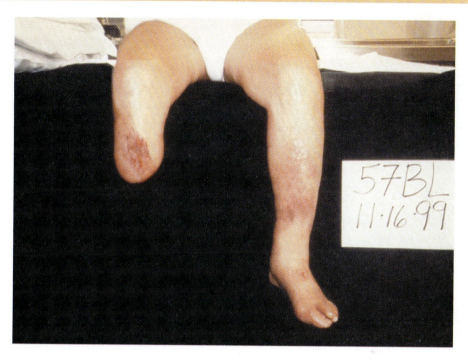

(Courtesy of Guthrie Healthcare System: Guthrie Lymphedema Clinic)

FIGURE 4-12c Secondary Lymphedema, Bilateral Lower Extremities

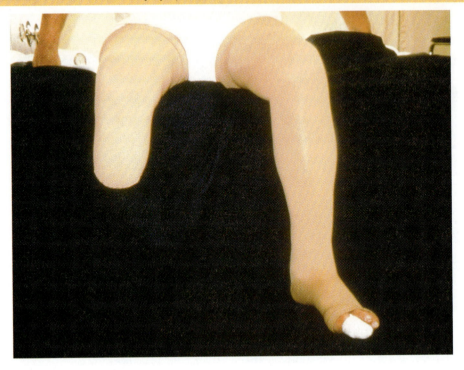

The patient has been fitted with compression garments at the end of Phase I, Treatment phase.
(Courtesy of Guthrie Healthcare System: Guthrie Lymphedema Clinic)

CASE 4–3 SECONDARY LYMPHEDEMA, MALIGNANT LYMPHEDEMA OF LEFT UPPER EXTREMITY

The patient, a 58-year-old female, was initially diagnosed with suspected left breast carcinoma. She initially presented with a palpable tumor in the left breast with skin ulceration, which had been present for quite some time before she consulted her physician. On March 10, 2000, the patient underwent a left modified radical mastectomy. The pathology report revealed benign breast tissue with five of the five axillary lymph nodes positive for metastasis. The subepidermal tissue demonstrated poorly differentiated carcinoma with skin ulceration and marked lymphovascular permeation. The tissue was a much higher grade than the typical breast carcinoma. Primary lung cancer was suspected as both glandular and squamous differentiation was suspected from the pathology report. Later, it was confirmed that the patient was suffering from NSCLC (non-small cell lung cancer). She was started on chemotherapy. No radiation followed the initial round of chemotherapy. A CT scan in May 2000 revealed multiple pulmonary nodules and extensive mediastinal adenopathy. Pericardial thickening was suggestive of pericardial metastasis. Swelling of the left arm initiated in May 2000 with rapid onset and associated pain.

The patient presented in our clinic August 25, 2000, approximately three months from the onset of symptoms. Using the formula for cone volume, it was estimated that the amount of edema present in the left arm was 116.5% larger than the right. There was 2637.19 mL of fluid volume. Height: 5 ft. 8 in.: Initial body weight: 183 lb.

Upon initial examination, the patient demonstrated minimal functional limitations. Skin ulcerations concentrated in the left anterior chest wall were deep-red clusters and no seepage was evident. The tissue throughout the left upper extremity was severely indurated. Pitting edema of 2+ was evident on the dorsum of the left hand.

Left upper extremity AROM was minimally limited and functional. She needed little assistance with dressing and was independent in grooming and transfers. She was able to drive to her appointments and was insistent on maintaining her independence as much as possible despite the 10/10 pain level. Her posture revealed a depressed left shoulder with a rounded posture and protracted scapula.

The patient was seen for a total of thirty treatment sessions of CDT. Treatment initiated on August 28, 2000 with immediate relief from pain within the first week of treatment. A decrease in the need for prescribed Percocet was reported at that time. Because of the difficulty with independent bandaging, use of an Arm-Assist® (a nonelastic limb containment system) was applied to assure continued independence with compression application. The device was highly effective. The patient was less dependent on her family, pain levels were reduced, and edema control was enhanced.

Ulcerations continued to invade the dermal tissue in the left upper arm, posterior trunk quadrant, and axilla. In October 2000, XRT was initiated to the area to control metastasis. On November 2, 2000, the patient was referred to the wound care center at the University of Pennsylvania for further progression of the skin lesions. Her skin regime consisted of Nystatin cream, Silvadene, Adaptic nonadhesive pads, and ABD pads. A home nurse followed skin care so that no dressing changes were necessary during her CDT sessions.

On a follow-up visit to the oncologist on November 27, 2000, it was reported that her CT scan on November 20, 2000 revealed continued aggressive disease. Tumors had become larger and spread to the left elbow. Bandaging was modified to the elbow on November 28, 2000, utilizing a 1/2-in. foam muff, dense foam on the dorsum of her hand, and short-stretch bandaging to assist with comfort. The limb containment system was no longer useful secondary to dermal ulceration throughout the upper arm. SOB pursued and general fatigue consumed her. CDT continued for palliation. The patient was last seen as an outpatient on January 2, 2001. One visit was made to the patient's home to offer support. She died on January 19, 2001.

The following measurements of volume and percentage of edema were tracked through seventeen treatment sessions. Following that time, the goals of treatment were readjusted and measurements were no longer documented.

	Volume (mL)	Edema (%)	Total reduction (%)
Initial Evaluation	2637.19	116.19	60.1
Week 1	1584.83	70.03	39.5
Week 2	1830.46	80.88	30.5
Week 3	1579.80	69.80	40.0
Week 4	1816.67	80.27	31.1
Week 5	1716.05	75.82	34.9
Week 6	1691.52	74.74	35.8
Week 7	1548.59	68.52	41.3

Measurements were discontinued following Week 7 secondary to the aggressive dermal ulcerations present throughout the left upper arm. Final weight was 162 lb. Functional level had dwindled to moderate assist with dressing and grooming. Pain levels initially dropped to 3/10 with a decrease in pain medication. Pain was never reported to the initial intensity in the left arm until a few weeks before the patient died. Towards the end of treatment, complaints of pain were mostly in the anterior chest, shoulder, and back. Constant compression via bandaging improved comfort levels as it served as a counterstimulus to pain sensations.

The challenges of providing CDT as an intervention for a person demonstrating malignant lymphedema are many. The patient may lack the strength, ROM, and motivation to comply with treatment responsibilities. In this particular case, malignant dermal invasion posed a significant challenge in finding healthy lymph pathways during MLD. The bandaging technique also had to be modified to accommodate the areas not affected. Because the disease involved the lungs, deep abdominal breathing became progressively difficult and triggered a distressing cough.

The family plays an integral part in the treatment phase of CDT. Bandaging instruction is essential and MLD techniques can be very helpful for the family and friends who are usually with the patient on a round-the-clock schedule. Involvement in the home program provides an opportunity for the loved ones to play an active role in the patient's care. Providing psychological and spiritual support for the patient is truly essential. It is important to develop an understanding of the benefits and challenges to providing care. Adapting treatment techniques and setting appropriate goals for this special population is an integral part of the therapist's responsibility. CDT proves valuable for the patient with advanced disease and will continue to be a necessary part of palliative lymphedema management. See Figures 4.13 a–b.

Submitted by Maureen Fleagle, PT, MLD/CDT, Penn Therapy and Fitness, University of Pennsylvania Health System.

FIGURE 4-13a Secondary Lymphedema, Upper Extremity at Initial Evaluation

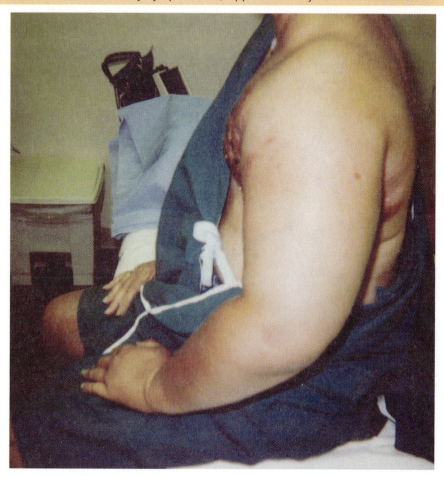

(Courtesy of Maureen Fleagle PT, MLD/CDT)

FIGURE 4-13b Secondary Lymphedema, Upper Extremity at the End of Palliative Intervention

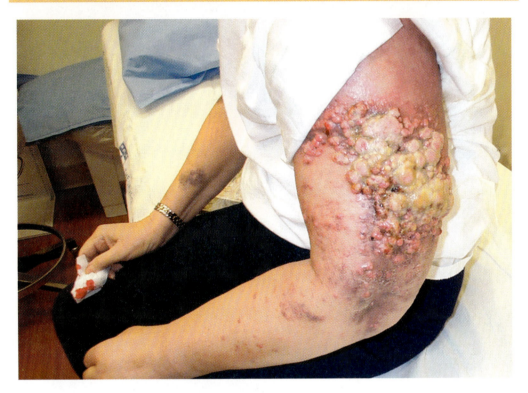

(Courtesy of Maureen Fleagle PT, MLD/CDT)

References

1. Franzeck, U. K., et al. 1997. Combined physical therapy for lymphedema evaluated by fluorescence microlymphography and lymph capillary pressure measurements. *J Vasc Res.* 34:306–11.

2. Hwang, J. H., et al. 1999. Changes in lymphatic function after complex physical therapy for lymphedema. *Lymphology* 32:15–21.

3. Rockson, et al. 1998. Workgroup III: Diagnosis and management of lymphedema. *Cancer* (Supplement) 83(12):2882–85.

4. Földi, E., Földi, M., Weissleder, H. 1985. Conservative treatment of lymphoedema of the limbs. *Angiology* 36(3):171–80.

5. Földi, E., Földi, M., Clodius, L. 1989. The lymphoedema chaos: A lancet. *Ann Plast Surg.* 22:505–15.

6. Casley-Smith, J. R. and Casley-Smith, J. R. 1992. Modern treatment for lymphoedema: Complex physical therapy: The first 200 Australian limbs. *Australas J Dermatol.* 33:61–68.

7. Mallon, E. C. and Ryan, T. J. 1994. Lymphedema and wound healing. *Clinics in Dermatology* 12:89–93.

8. Ko, D., Lerner, R., Klose, G., Cosimi, A. B. 1998. Effective treatment of lymphedema of the extremities. *Arch Surg.* 133:452–58.

9. Casley-Smith, J. R. 1983. Varying total tissue pressures and the concentration of initial lymphatic lymph. *Microvascular Research* 25:369–79.

10. Mortimer, P. S., et al. 1990. The measurement of skin lymph flow by isotope clearance-reliability, reproducibility, injection dynam-

ics and the effect of massage. *J Invest Dermatol.* 95(6):677–82.

11. Olszewski, W. L. and Engeset, A. 1980. Intrinsic contractility of prenodal lymph vessels and lymph flow in human leg. *Am J Physiol.* 239(6):H775–83.

12. Smith, A. 1987. Lymphatic drainage in patients after replantation of extremities. *Plast Reconstr Surg.* 79:163–68.

13. Hutzschenreuter, P., Brummer, H., Ebberfeld, K. 1989. Experimental and clinical studies of the mechanism of effect of manual lymph drainage therapy. *Z Lymphol.* 13(1):62–64. (Article in German.)

14. Eliska, O. and Eliskova, M. 1995. Are peripheral lymphatics damaged by high pressure manual massage? *Lymphology* 28:21–30.

15. Leduc, O., Peeters, A., Borgeois, P. 1990. Bandages: Scintigraphic demonstration of its efficacy on colloidal protein reabsorption during muscle activity. *Progress in Lymphology-XII.* Elsevier Science Publishers.

16. Johansson, K., Albertsson, M., Ingvar, C., Ekdahl, C. 1999. Effects of compression bandaging with or without manual lymph drainage treatment in patients with postoperative arm lymphedema. *Lymphology* 32:103–10.

17. Schmid-Schönbein, G. W. 1990. Microlymphatics and lymph flow. *Physiol Rev.* 70(4):987–1028.

18. Brennan, M. J., DePompolo, R. W., Garden, F. H. 1996. Focused review: Postmastectomy lymphedema. *Arch Phys Med Rehabil.* 77:S-74-S-80.

19. Badger, C. M., Peacock, J. L., Mortimer, P. S. 2000. A randomized, controlled, parallel-group clinical trial comparing multilayer bandaging followed by hosiery versus hosiery alone in the treatment of patients with lymphedema of the limb. *Cancer* 88(12):2832–37.

20. Hutzschenreuter, P. and Brummer, H. 1986. Lymphangiomotoricity and tissue pressure. *Z Lymphol.* 10(2):55–57. (Article in German.)

21. Stemmer, R., Marescaux, J., Furderer, C. 1980. Compression therapy of the lower extremities particulary with compression stockings.

Hautarzt (Dermatologist) 31:355–65. (Article in German.)

22. Weissleder, H. and Schuchhardt, C. 1997. *Lymphedema Diagnosis and Therapy*, 2nd ed. Bonn: Kagerer Kommunication.

23. Lerner, R. 1998. What's new in lymphedema therapy in America? *International Journal of Angiology* 7:191–96.

24. Wittlinger, H. 1989. *Textbook of Dr. Vodder's Manual Lymphatic Drainage II.* Heidelberg, Germany: Karl R. Hang Publishers.

25. Dimeo, F. C., Tilmann, M. H., Bertz, H., Kanz, L., et al. 1997. Aerobic exercise in the rehabilitation of cancer patients after high dose chemotherapy and autologous peripheral stem cell transplantation. *Cancer* 79(9):1717–22.

26. Graydon, J. E., Bubela, N., Irvine, D., Vincent, L. 1995. Fatigue-reducing strategies used by patients receiving treatment for cancer. *Cancer Nurs.* 18(1):23–28.

27. Piller, N. B. 1976. Conservative treatment of acute and chronic lymphoedema with benzo-pyrones. *Lymphology* 9:132–37.

28. Földi, M. 1998. Are there enigmas concerning the pathophysiology of lymphedema after breast cancer treatment? *NLN Newsletter.* 10(4):1–4.

29. 1997. *Designing Resistance Training Programs*, 2nd ed. Fleck, S. J. and Kraemer, W. J. eds. Chicago: Human Kinetics.

30. Lewis, C. B., Bottomley, J. M. 1994. *Geriatric Physical Therapy—A Clinical Approach.* Norwalk, CT: Appleton & Lange.

31. Harris, S. R. and Niesen-Vertommen, S. L. 2000. Challenging the myth of exercise-induced lymphedema following breast cancer: A series of case reports. *J Surg Oncol.* 74:95–99.

32. Yasuhara, H., Shigematsu, H., Muto, T. 1996. A study of the advantages of elastic stockings for leg lymphedema. *Int Angiol.* 15(3):272–77.

33. Rudkin, G. and Miller, T. 1994. Lipedema: A clinical entity distinct from lymphedema. *Plastic and Reconstructive Surgery* 94(6): 841–47; discussion 848–49.

5

OTHER INTERVENTION OPTIONS

"... while we can recommend the best possible regime, it is a regime and the patients are the ones who have to live with it."

JUDITH AND JOHN CASLEY-SMITH,
PIONEERS IN LYMPHEDEMA RESEARCH AND PATIENT CARE

INTRODUCTION

In addition to CDT, there are a variety of both historical and new treatments available for use in intervention plans for lymphedema management. Delivery of the techniques and evaluation of the scientific literature, however, should be examined in light of current knowledge of the anatomic and physiologic principles of the lymph system.

THE PNEUMATIC COMPRESSION PUMP

The compression pump is a pneumatic unit designed to apply external pressure to an extremity. The unit consists of a sleeve to fit either an upper or lower extremity, and a device for pumping air into the sleeve through rubber tubing. Appliances come in a variety of styles with variable settings. Controls can adjust the amount of pressure and the timing of the on and off cycles. Some sleeves have cells or chambers that fill segmentally or sequentially.

The practice of using the compression pump to treat lymphedema has evolved slowly beginning in the 1950s. Interested readers should refer to the comprehensive historical overview by Augustine,[1] which outlines the history of the pump, the paradigm shift in treatment, and the ongoing investigation among management experts and researchers into how and when the compression pump should be used in the treatment of lymphedema.

Historically, the compression pump has been used most often for lower extremity treatment to prevent deep vein thrombosis and pulmonary embolism as well as to improve the return of venous blood from an extremity back into general circulation. During the 1950s attention was turned to the use of the compression pump to treat lymphedema. Since that time clinical and research activities surrounding the pump have produced variable data: numerous complications have been documented, new types of compression pumps have been designed, and literature supporting and opposing the use of pumps has been published. Guidelines for pump selection and use are unclear.[2] In the literature, no certain pump, or style of pump, appears to be more effective than another.[3–6]

For years, the compression pump was the "treatment of choice" for lymphedema therapy in North America. It was thought that the compression device could imitate the mechanical effects of massage. The setting for delivery of this treatment has varied based on the education and opinion of the referring practitioner. Some patients receive compression treatment in occupational or physical therapy clinics, some are sent directly to a medical supply vendor with a prescription to rent or purchase a pump. The instructions and guidelines for use, which the patient is likely to receive, are also variable. Patients and clinicians alike are seeking current information on how and when to use the pump most safely and effectively.

Opinions vary as to the safety, efficacy, and utility of the compression pump. Many management experts from around the world do not support use of the compression pump for the majority of patients with lymphedema. "These pumps are of limited value in the early stages of lymphedema and virtually useless in later stages."[7] "To squeeze edema fluid towards the groin or axilla of a lymphedematous limb, especially if the regional lymph nodes have been removed or are diseased, defies an understanding of basic anatomy and physiology."[8] "Unfortunately, the experience of using a pneumatic pump is uniformly dismal in the treatment of lymphedema; therefore, in our opinion, it should not be recommended as an effective form of therapy."[9] "Although the use of machinery for the pumping action on the arm lymphatics is theoretically attractive, pumping has not been as effective clinically as had been hoped."[10] "We demonstrated that intermittent compression has a limited role in the treatment of postmastectomy lymphedema."[11]

Other investigators, primarily surgeons, indicate findings that support use of the pump.[12-14] Many studies that support the use of the pump are small, only one published randomized clinical trial exists and only a few follow subjects long term for possible existence of exacerbations. Most investigators who support use of the pump now recommend the pump as part of a comprehensive intervention plan, which includes MLD, lymphedema bandaging, exercise, skin care, and compression garments.

Despite support from some health care professionals for the continued use of this type of intervention, treatment parameters have yet to be agreed on. Both opinions and evidence vary concerning amount of pressure, length and frequency of each treatment session, duration of treatment over time, and type of machine (single chamber vs multichamber). In addition to confusion surrounding treatment protocol, potential complications resulting from the use of the compression pump to treat lymphedema may outweigh potential benefits.[15] (See pages 105–106.) Compression provided by a machine is generalized, does not remove protein and does not have a significant clinical effect on fibrotic tissues.[7,14] In contrast, manual techniques can deliver delicate and specific varying pressures, soften excess fibrosis, and remove protein.[16,17]

One of the prevailing themes of this text is the challenge to measure all interventions against what is currently known about the anatomy and physiology of the lymphatic system. Although the healing effects of compression, particulary for the lower extremities, have been accepted since ancient times, our understanding of human microcirculation has grown significantly in the last 50 years. In keeping with the theme, this chapter will examine the potential effects of the pneumatic pump and suggest an intervention scheme based on current knowledge.

It is clear that during pumping, the majority of the fluid moved from the interstitium into the venous system is water.[18-23] Most of the reduction achieved will occur because fluid (primarily water) is forced into blood capillaries.[24] Recall from Chapters 1 through 4 that protein molecules, which are left behind when water is mechanically forced out of the interstitium, will attract more water to the area unless they are effectively removed as well. To achieve maximum fluid and protein removal by the lymphatic system, the treatment selected must not only raise tissue hydrostatic pressure but also vary that pressure as much as possible. To avoid collapse of the initial lymphatics, tissue pressure must simultaneously be mild.[24–26] To assure long-term results, intervention should also include treatment features that will enhance the possibility of increasing and/or altering lymph flow patterns to take advantage of anastomoses. Rerouting around scar tissue and mobilizing fluid uptake using remaining viable lymphatics will also facilitate long-term resolution.

A SUGGESTED APPROACH TO THE USE OF THE PNEUMATIC PUMP

Appropriate patient selection:

- **The patient who cannot or will not tolerate lymphedema bandaging.** Careful use of the pump along with MLD and the other components of CDT may lead to a successful outcome. There are, however, a number of static compression devices that may better meet the needs of this patient. See "Alternative compression therapy options" on page 106 and refer to Chapter 8 for a comprehensive list of vendors.
- **The patient with minimal fibrotic changes to subcutaneous tissues.** Clinically, this is determined with history, palpation, observation, and occasionally with the use of tonometry.
- **The patient who cannot come for daily treatment** may be able to supplement treatment with a compression pump at some point in the intervention plan.

Machine features:

- *Sequential pumping action.* Since lymph vessel valves are often incompetent in lymphedema, it is best, if any pump is used, to use a sequential pump for treatment. A pump that compresses the entire limb at once will promote minimal lymph flow. The most distal portion of the appliance sleeve should deliver the greatest pressure during treatment, with the most proximal end delivering minimal pressure.
- *Compression settings that can be adjusted at or near 0 mm Hg.* The pressure during the rest cycle should be as low as possible to allow refilling of vessels. The 0 mm Hg pressure setting is optimal.
- *On–off cycle settings in increments of seconds (not limited to increments of minutes).* Based on the pulsation rate of lymphatic vessels, and normal emptying and filling times, the best interval for compression and relaxation is measured in seconds. Existing pumps often have a slower frequency and do not offer a 5-second rest cycle. If use of the pump is justified, the appropriate style is one that allows short rest and short compression cycles.
- *Appliance sleeve with narrow compression segments (or cells).* For maximal flow out of the regions that have just been compressed, the compressing segments of the sleeve should be as narrow as possible. Initial studies show that segments within the appliance sleeve appear to be optimal if they are approximately 3 cm wide.[27]
- One example of a device that fits the description above fairly closely is the *Lympha Press®*. Refer to Chapter 8 for details about distribution.

Machine settings for treatment:

- Based on tissue hydrostatic pressure, total tissue pressure, and lymph flow, pressure settings that may not hinder lymphatic system function can be calculated for machines. The best pressure settings will be 45 mm Hg and lower.[27] Some investigators have used very high compression settings in controlled studies but little has been recorded about the long-term effects to the limb or the potential trauma to existing vessels.
- *Compression cycle (On)* = 30 seconds
- *Rest cycle (Off)* = 5 seconds upper extremity, 10 seconds lower extremity. A 5-second rest cycle for the arm and a 10-second rest cycle for the leg is adequate to allow relaxation and filling of lymphatics after emptying.[27]
- *Pressure* during compression cycle should not exceed 45 mm Hg. Since lymphatic vessel collapse occurs at pressures greater than 60 mm Hg,[24,26,28] avoid the application of greater pressures. Begin with a pressure setting of 20 mm Hg. Decrease the setting if any complications arise. (See Precautions and Contraindications on page 105.) Increase up to a maximum of 45 mm Hg at subsequent treatment sessions if limb reductions occur without complications.
- *Total treatment time* Start with 20 minutes, closely monitor patient reactions. Wait 24 hours and re-evaluate the patient for adverse reactions. If no complications arise, add 10 minutes each day, up to a treatment time of one hour. If patient response remains positive, add a second one-hour session to each day. Add the second hour in increments of 10 minutes, monitoring patient reactions closely.

Use safely:

- Anticipate potential problems and screen for them at each treatment session.
- Use sequential style pump, low pressures, short cycles, short overall treatment time.
- As with all applications of the compression pump, apply a layer of clean stockinette over the limb to be treated before applying the appliance sleeve. For the patient with lymphedema, a refined fabric such as *tg Stockinette* made by Lohmann or *Tricofix®* made by BSN-Jobst will provide needed protection for the limb surface. See Chapter 8 for product information.
- As agreed at the 1993 International Congress of Lymphology, if pumps are used at all, the "body reservoirs" should be cleared first.[29] This means that specific manual techniques should be used to increase lymphatic flow and emptying of vessels in the area of the trunk adjacent to the affected limb, as well as the base of the limb itself. These techniques are taught in specific education programs for CDT. See Chapter 8.
- Empty ipsilateral, contralateral, and trunk lymph nodes manually every 5 to 10 minutes during treatment.
- Patients must have adequate cognitive skills or family support to monitor for signs and symptoms of complications.
- Educate patient about precautions and instruct in manual emptying of lymph nodes and vessels as appropriate.
- Individualize a program based on what works best for each patient.

Precautions:
- Changes to treated limb: Numbness, tingling, redness, pain, decrease in joint range of motion after treatment, skin breakdown.
- Lymphatic vessels become dilated or visible during or after treatment (indicates blockage).
- Increase in swelling proximal to appliance sleeve (including genital area and breast region).
- Changes in skin texture at the base of the limb, which could indicate the formation of a fibrotic "cuff." The "cuff" may be due to congestion of lymph as it is forced to the base of the limb but is unable to exit the region due to decreased or absent lymphatic function.[30]

Contraindications:
- Brachial plexus lesions (Any pressure is contraindicated.)
- Radical breast surgery with radiation (Scarring and fibrosis are not effectively treated with compression pump.)
- Bilateral mastectomy (Fluid must be rerouted manually across the back and toward the lower trunk.)
- S/P Pelvic surgery if proximal portions of the lower extremities have begun to swell (Pump application will worsen symptoms.)
- Primary lymphedema (A clinically normal, contralateral (opposite) extremity often has abnormal drainage and preclinical lymphedema. There is significant potential for swelling to appear in adjacent quadrants.)
- More than one area of the body involved (primary or secondary)
- Swelling present in abdomen or genitalia (Crucial but challenging-to-treat areas of central drainage must be kept open.)
- Lymphatic vessels are dilated and visible prior to treatment (Indicates blockage.)
- Compression is contraindicated for lower extremities at an ABI <0.8. See Chapter 3 for a description of this noninvasive assessment of lower extremity circulation.
- Deep vein thrombosis
- Infection in the limb to be treated
- Malignancy in the limb to be treated or proximal to the limb
- Patients taking anticoagulant therapy (Work closely with referring practitioner.)
- Ongoing radiation therapy (RT) for active cancer in the limb or surrounding area
- Renal insufficiency, cardiac insufficiency, hypertension (Select a more controlled form of fluid reduction.)

Relative Advantages:
- A reduction in edema may help lymphatics to pump more effectively
- Harmful effects of swelling may be decreased locally
- Can be used at home (Patient should be closely supervised at each treatment until all pump settings, signs and symptoms of complications, and adjacent quadrant clearing have been mastered by the patient.)

Disadvantages:

- Lengthy treatment time (Some protocols suggest up to 8 hours/day)
- Patient immobility during treatment
- Complaints of pain (by some patients) when limb is compressed even at low pressures
- Risk of previously clear, adjacent trunk quadrant filling with fluid
- Cost of machine to purchase or rent (Potential waste if treatment is not effective.)
- Risk of symptom exacerbation
- Risk of onset of genital swelling and/or pelvic congestion with lower extremity treatment[31]
- Risk of trauma to residual, functioning lymph vessels by pressures applied
- Lack of strong support from management experts and the literature

The majority of evidence including statistical details, alterations in lymph transport capacity, and amounts of tissue proteins favors manual methods of intervention. If chosen as part of the intervention plan, the compression pump should be used selectively and cautiously with constant monitoring by the patient and therapist for complications. *When used, the pump should not be used alone but should be an adjunct to other intervention.* Clinician knowledge of specific manual techniques is needed to safely reduce risk of complications from compression pump treatments.

COMPRESSION GARMENTS

In addition to coverage of the compression garment in Chapter 4, a short discussion is included here because, historically, part of the North American treatment regime has been use of the garment as the first or only intervention. The premature application of stockings or sleeves before the bulk of edema fluid had been properly evacuated was a widely practiced method, which indicated a lack of understanding of lymphatic anatomy and physiology.[8] It is not helpful to fit compression garments before beginning volume-reducing techniques.[32,33] The effect of compressive or constrictive pressures on lymph flow are discussed in Chapter 1. In addition to the negative influences on circulation, there are resulting issues of discomfort to address. Patients who are fitted with a garment before adequate treatment has reduced their swelling frequently report that the garment is uncomfortable at best. This common complaint translates into poor adherence with garment wear among those who are trying to tolerate the garment over a limb which has not been adequately reduced. At this point patients also complain of chafing marks, skin breakdown, pain, and an increase in swelling of adjacent areas. Application of the garment after limb reduction is compatible with lymphatic anatomy and physiology will conserve limb reduction and skin health changes, and improve the likelihood of patient satisfaction and adherence to the compression garment portion of the self-management phase.

ALTERNATIVE COMPRESSION THERAPY OPTIONS

There are a variety of nonelastic limb containment systems/compression aids on the market. The designers and distributors state that these devices are intended to support or replace the use of lymphedema bandaging. Application of lymphedema bandaging is more customized to the individual limb and allows for unlimited modifications. A limb

FIGURE 5-1 Example of a Pneumatic Compression Device

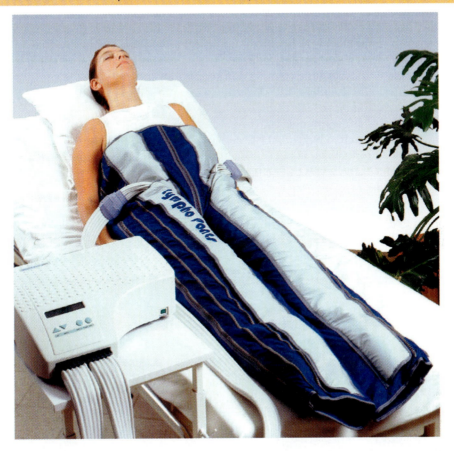

The Lympha Press® overlapping pants which cover the groin area as well as the lower extremities.
(Courtesy of Mego Afek Instruments, Medical Division)

containment system, however, may be appropriate during or after a course of CDT if the patient is unable to use lymphedema bandaging due to lack of family support, limitations in hand function needed to bandage, visual or cognitive limitations, or difficulty bending to reach lower extremities. Some of these devices work well in combination with a compression garment in the self-management phase. This combination may work well for the individual with lower extremity lymphedema who stands a lot during the day.

Typically, a prescription for a compression garment is required to obtain these devices. They can range from $200 US to $900 US depending on the style and features selected. Some of the systems must be replaced every six months, while others may last up to two years. As always, check the literature for support of current compression theories and appraise the value of the device in light of its compatibility with the functions of the lymphatic system and the needs of the patient. Refer to Chapter 8 for information on how to contact the individual companies.

- *ReidSleeve®*: Manufactured by Peninsula Medical, Inc., the patented ReidSleeve® applies pressure using a foam insert and adjustable straps. A patented gauge is used to assess the pressure over any region of the limb contained in the sleeve. Patients can fit the sleeve without assistance. The sleeve can be adjusted as limb reduction occurs. Styles available through Peninsula Medical include compression support for the upper and lower extremities. The ReidSleeve® is typically worn at night in place of bandaging. See Figure 5.2.
- *CircAid©:* A variety of upper and lower extremity compression systems are made and distributed by CircAid© Medical Products. Materials include adjustable, interlocking, nonelastic bands that are tightened around a foam liner. Compression levels can be monitored in the upper extremity system. See Figure 5.3.
- *Arm Assist®/Leg Assist®:* These compression sleeves are made and distributed by MedAssist-OP, Inc. They are custom-fabricated based on measurements taken by the clinician. The strapping system can be adjusted

FIGURE 5-2 Upper Extremity Application of the ReidSleeve Classic®

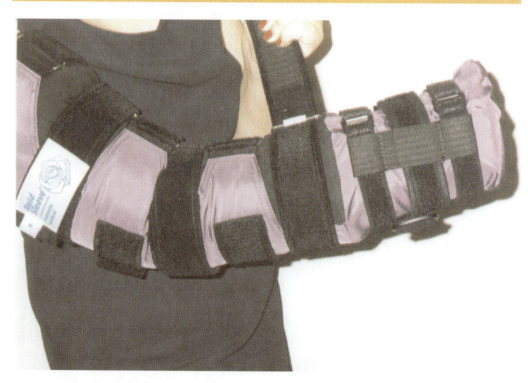

An example of a nonelastic limb containment system.

(Courtesy of Peninsula Medical, Inc.)

FIGURE 5-3 Upper Extremity Application of the CircAid® Measure-Up™

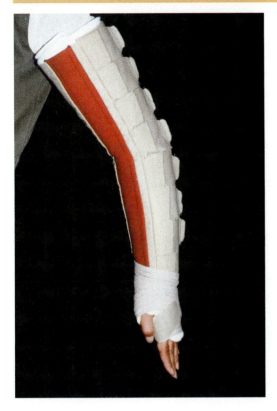

An example of a nonelastic limb containment system.

(Courtesy of CircAid Medical Products, Inc.)

with one hand. Styles include options for the upper and lower extremities. See Figure 5.4.

KINESIO TAPING® METHOD WITH KINESIO® TEX TAPE

Initiated in 1973 by Kenzo Kase, D.C., the Kinesio Taping® Method is a treatment that is purported to effect the neurological, musculoskeletal, and circulatory systems. It is used to treat a variety of diagnoses including lymphedema. The method includes specific taping techniques applied to involved body regions with specially created Kinesio® Tex Tape. The tape is highly elastic, latex, and zinc free. It has been suggested that the taping method may provide skin movement through traction and may also affect tissue pressures. Both of these responses have been shown, in other unrelated studies, to alter lymphatic fluid movement.[34] One investigator found the taping method was effective in softening fibrotic areas of soft tissue.[35] Another study states that blood flow is increased in the specifically treated body area following application of the taping method.[36] While significant numbers of controlled studies are lacking, the taping method and taping products have found a place in the list of lymphedema intervention options. It has been suggested that the taping procedure is best used during the manual therapy portion of the intervention.

The taping method will be described in detail in two textbooks to be published in the near future.[a,b] Additionally, instruction in the taping method has been instituted in all recertification courses for participants in the Vodder School of North America,

FIGURE 5-4 Upper Extremity Application of the ArmAssist™

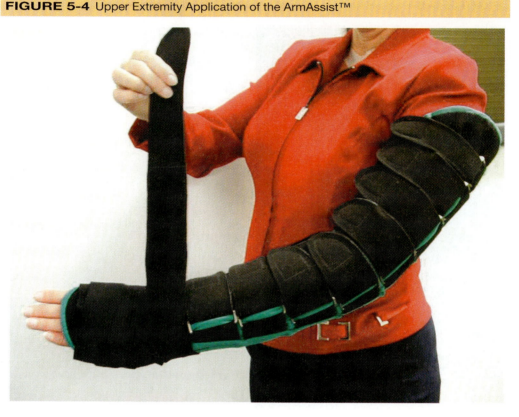

An example of a nonelastic limb containment system.
(Courtesy of MedAssist -OP, Inc.)

which provides specific education in lymphedema management. See Chapter 8 for contact information.

SURGICAL THERAPY

Surgical procedures have been used extensively for the past century to treat lymphedema. Many different types of procedures have been attempted, yet none has been consistently clinically successful.[10,37] Currently, a curative surgical technique is not available. Many surgeons concur that surgical therapy should only be used after an aggressive trial of medical management has failed.[13,38] Surgery would most likely be indicated if vision was compromised due to facial swelling or if genitourinary function is affected. Management experts maintain that a course of CDT achieves similar or better results with no risk to the patient and at less cost.[7,9] All this being said, many surgeons are still suggesting surgical therapy for the management of their patients with chronic lymphedema. The types of surgery fit into two primary categories outlined as follows. Potential complications appear across all types of surgery.[4,7,9,10,38,39]

[a]*Rehabilitation of the Hand,* Callahan and Malick. To be published by Mosby—2001.
[b]*Splinting the Upper Extremity,* Jacobs and Austin. To be published by Lippincott, Wilkins & Williams—2001.

FIGURE 5-5 Kinesio® Tex Tape Products

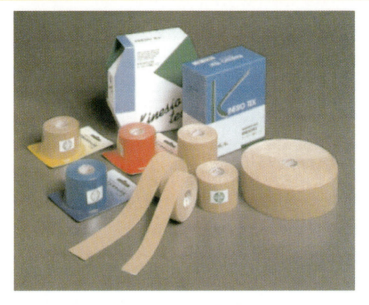

(Courtesy of Kinesio USA, 1100S Spain NE #2, Albuquerque, NM 87111)

Debulking/excisional or reduction surgery

Reduction approaches remove subcutaneous fat and lymphedematous tissue. The excised area is covered with a skin graft. This type of surgery does not improve drainage of lymph but reduces the amount of tissue in which edema may develop.

- The *Charles Procedure* is an example of a debulking technique. First described in 1912, it is still in use today despite significant complications.[39]
- *Liposuction* is another example of a debulking technique. Still controversial, there are several groups studying the effects of carefully controlled liposuction. Long-term efficacy is not known.[39,40,41] Most of the current results from liposuction involve the use of MLD and compression garments in addition to the surgical technique.[41] It should be noted that fatty tissue cannot be removed without disturbing local microcirculation. The long-term impact on the remaining lymphatic system has not been investigated except in the animal model. Some clinicians report a small patient population now emerging with lymphedema of the lower extremities following liposuction of the abdominal area for cosmetic purposes.

Physiologic/functional surgery

Physiologic approaches attempt to enhance lymphatic function. Lymphatic channels are reconstructed, or microsurgical anastomoses are made from one lymphatic vessel to another lymphatic vessel, or lymphatic vessels to veins. One of the greatest challenges for surgeons is how to facilitate a successful anastomosis at the juncture of lymph vessel, where fluid flows at a lower pressure, and a vein where fluid flows at a higher pressure. An artificially created anastomosis may fail due to the pressure differential at the surgical connection.

- The *microlymphatic-venous anastomosis (LVA)* is an example of a physiologic procedure. Results have been positive for some patients but the number of patients studied was small.
- The *lymphatic-venous-lymphatic (LVL) interpositioned grafted shunt* is another example of a physiologic procedure. Results have been positive for some patients but again the number of patients studied was small.[42]

Complications (Surgical morbidity)
- Skin necrosis—particulary in the area of skin graft with the debulking procedures (23% incidence)[13]
- Regression to preoperative size or larger[14]
- Slow healing of surgical wounds[7]
- Damage to or removal of functioning lymphatics through dissection or liposuction
- Postoperative infection
- Potential need for multiple procedures[7,38,39,42]

NUTRITION THERAPY

There is no known diet or food supplement that has been proven to safely decrease the signs and symptoms of lymphedema. There are individuals interested in exploring the possibility of using over-the-counter herbal supplements such as grape seed extract or bioflavonoids to alter the body's response to swelling. As with all nonregulated supplements, individuals should exercise caution when ingesting these, especially in large quantities. Individuals with lymphedema who wish to try dietary alterations or food supplements to effect swelling should work closely with a physician educated in the anatomy and physiology of the lymphatic system. Eating well to control body weight and promote overall good health is recommended. As seen in the general population, a low-salt, low-fat diet may contribute to weight control.

DRUG THERAPY

- *Benzopyrones:* A group of drugs called benzopyrones have been shown both clinically and experimentally to assist in the reduction of the signs and symptoms of lymphedema. This group of drugs includes flavonoids and coumarin (not to be confused with the prescription drug called *Coumadin*™). Benzopyrones stimulate macrophage activity, which increases proteolysis. Remember from Chapters 1 and 2 that excess protein in the tissue spaces leads to decreased oncotic pressure in plasma and increased fluid collection. The normal process of deposition and lysis of collagen fibers is disrupted—with more deposition than lysis occurring, leading to fibrosis. Researchers have used benzopyrones to treat lymphedema clinically and experimentally for over 20 years in Europe and Australia. [43–46] Results indicate a slow reduction in signs and symptoms of lymphedema, which is further enhanced when the drugs are used orally and/or topically in conjunction with other intervention such as CDT. It can take six months or more to notice the effects of the drug.[45] Patients must take the drug indefinitely to maintain the effects.

The benzopyrones may cause liver toxicity, however, and deaths have been reported. In a recent study in North America, benzopyrones showed no value beyond the placebo effect.[47] In the United States, several benzopyrones are used clinically but none have been approved by the FDA. As of press time, a number of studies related to the use of benzopyrones are under way in North America and may be published in the near future. Both the National Lymphedema Network and the National Alliance of Breast Cancer Organizations (NABCO) strongly advise patients **not** to take benzopyrones outside of a clinical trial setting. Names of benzopyrones, which you will see in the literature, include but are not limited to *Venalot*[TM], *Paroven, Venoruton, Relvène, Endotélon,*[TM] and *Daflon.*

- *Diuretics:* This group of drugs has long been used in an attempt to address peripheral edema of all types, including lymphedema. While attractive as a potential solution to swelling, a review of their action in the body causes most management experts to shun their use. Diuretics indirectly lower microvascular hydrostatic pressure by plasma volume contraction.[48] A decrease in fluid, without the removal of the lingering protein molecules, will give temporary results before triggering a rapid return of fluid to the area.[49] Patients with comorbidities may be at risk of other health complications with the introduction of diuretics.

Clinical implications: It is important to note during the history portion of an examination whether the patient has received previous treatments with a compression pump, alternative compression therapy aids, a compression garment, and drug or surgical therapy. Information about patient response to these treatments as well as a thorough examination of the skin near the base of the "previously treated" limb will assist in planning intervention.

SUMMARY

Many patients, clinicians, and referring practitioners are looking for quick and easy ways to manage the signs and symptoms of lymphedema. The term *quick and easy* is not always synonymous with the most effective and biocompatible forms of intervention. Historically, most ailing body systems require time to repair themselves. The best intervention is often that which facilitates the body's own response to healing. Even CDT, thought by many to be the most effective treatment, is reported to remove only about 50% of the fluid per year.[50,51] Another year is required before tissue remodeling will allow much more to be removed.[45] Early, accurate diagnosis, along with early and appropriate intervention, are crucial to timely, positive results.

When planning any type of intervention strategy, consider:

- compatibility with anatomy and physiology (gentle to intact superficial vessels, assists in dispersal of accumulated interstitial protein)
- safety
- cost—short and long term
- comfort
- patient satisfaction, adherence, and quality of life issues
- short-term physiological effects
- long-term physiological effects

CASE STUDIES

CASE 5–1 PRIMARY LYMPHEDEMA, RIGHT LOWER EXTREMITY

PM was a 55-year-old male with a PMH of left AKA at age 4, following traumatic event. Swelling began in right lower extremity at age 53: insidious onset. Initially, through another health care setting, the patient used a compression pump for 3 days, 45 minutes per day. Lower extremity swelling increased and included genital swelling. One- and-one-half years after onset of swelling, the patient presented to our clinic unable to wear left leg prosthesis secondary to genital swelling. Patient reported pain in scrotum as 5/10 on a visual analog pain scale. Patient was using axillary crutches and wheelchair for mobility. Treatment consisted of five-part CDT program, as well as skin care for the genital area. Skin care included application of petroleum jelly and Adaptic dressing covered by 4×4s, Kerlix, and ABD pads to control drainage. Genital dressings were anchored around the waist using Idealbinde®, Kerlix, and Coban. Thirty treatments were administered over six weeks. The patient and his spouse continue to wrap the genital region at home, following techniques used during treatment. The patient was fitted with a thigh-high stocking, Class 3 (40–50 mm Hg) compression gradient.

See Figures 5.6a and b.

Measurements in centimeters		
Right lower extremity		
	4/12/99	5/28/00
MT base	30.0	26.5
4 cm above	32.7	27.0
8 cm above	34.5	29.0
Malleoli	44.5	31.0
4 cm above	53.9	32.5
8 cm above	57.0	36.0
12 cm	60.3	44.0
16 cm	63.7	47.0
20 cm	69.7	47.0
24 cm	72.5	49.5
28 cm	72.0	48.5
32 cm	71.0	48.0
36 cm	65.5	49.0
40 cm	64.0	48.5
44 cm	63.5	52.5
48 cm	68.5	53.5
52 cm	70.5	56.0
56 cm	71.5	61.0
Scrotum	51.5	34.0 (middle circumference)

FIGURE 5-6a Primary Lymphedema of the Right Lower Extremity and Genitalia before Intervention

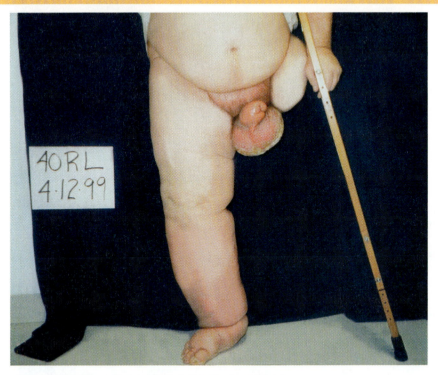

(Courtesy of Guthrie Healthcare System: Guthrie Lymphedema Clinic)

FIGURE 5-6b Primary Lymphedema of the Right Lower Extremity and Genitalia after Complete Decongestive Therapy (CDT)

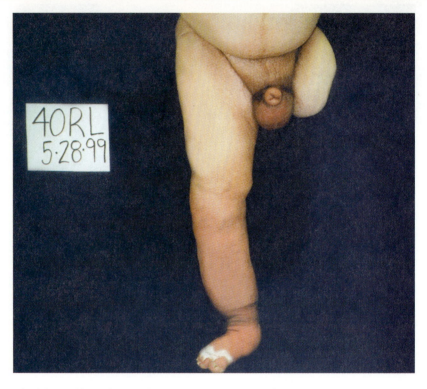

(Courtesy of Guthrie Healthcare System: Guthrie Lymphedema Clinic)

CASE 2   PRIMARY LYMPHEDEMA (TARDA), LEFT LOWER EXTREMITY

HP is a 63-year-old male s/p MVA with left ankle sprain in 1975. His lower extremity was swollen following the accident and did not subside for 25 years. The patient also sustained left foot drop following MVA. CDT was initiated 1/17/00. Patient was seen 5 days/week for 25 visits. Lymphedema bandaging included Komprex® high-density foam and Schneider packs (see Chapter 8 for descriptions of these bandaging additions). Following Phase I, the patient was fitted with a thigh-high compression garment, Class 3 (40–50 mm Hg) compression gradient, with an open toe design. He was also fitted with a nonelastic limb containment system and a custom AFO, both to be worn over his compression stocking while at work during Phase II of CDT.

See Figures 5.7a and b.

Measurements in centimeters		
Left lower extremity		
	1/17/00	2/17/00
MT base	25.0	21.5
4 cm above	28.0	22.4
8 cm above	29.5	24.5
Malleoli	35.0	25.5
4 cm above	36.0	23.5
8 cm above	40.4	25.6
12 cm	44.0	28.5
16 cm	47.5	32.1
20 cm	49.5	34.0
24 cm	49.5	35.2
28 cm	48.5	36.1
32 cm	46.0	37.0
36 cm	44.5	39.5
40 cm	47.5	41.5
44 cm	49.0	44.8
48 cm	51.3	48.0
52 cm	54.0	52.0
56 cm	57.0	55.3
60 cm	60.0	57.0
64 cm	62.0	60.0

Case studies 1 and 2 were submitted by Barbara Ann De Olden Murphy MSPT, MLD/CDT and Carrie Sullivan PTA, MLD/CDT, Guthrie Lymphedema Clinic; Guthrie Healthcare Systems, Sayre, PA.

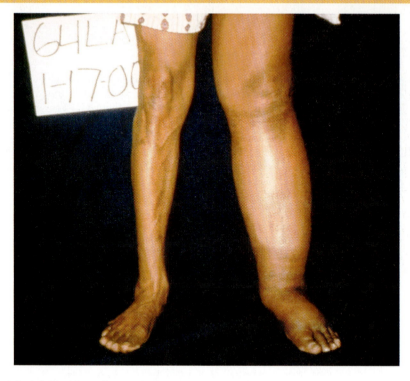

(Courtesy of Guthrie Healthcare System: Guthrie Lymphedema Clinic)

FIGURE 5-7b Primary Lymphedema of the Left Lower Extremity, after Complete Decongestive Therapy (CDT)

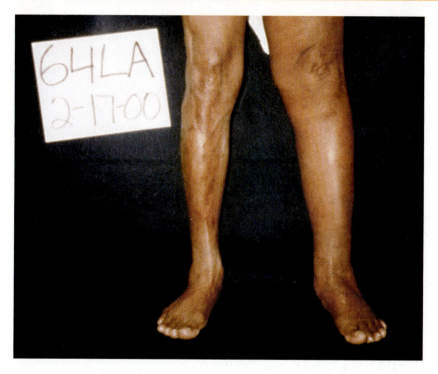

(Courtesy of Guthrie Healthcare System: Guthrie Lymphedema Clinic)

CASE 3   PATIENT PROFILE

The patient is a 57-year-old right-handed female who underwent a left modified radical mastectomy in 1983. She subsequently underwent a right modified radical mastectomy in 1991. She had no chemotherapy or radiation at either time. Patient reports she had since returned to full activity, including a regular exercise program, with no limitations.

The patient reported that in August 1997, she experienced a sharp pain in her right forearm after helping her husband move some heavy furniture. The pain in her forearm increased over the next several days and she noticed increased difficulty with elbow extension and wrist extension secondary to the increased pain. It was also at that time that she noticed slight swelling around her wrist and distal forearm. Since that time, the edema has gotten "minimally better" but the pain has persisted and continues to limit her activity. She notes that the edema "seems to worsen" with attempts at increased activity.

The patient reports going for a physical therapy consult during which time she was fitted for a compression sleeve. It was also recommended to her that she obtain a compression pump for home use. She did not choose to follow up with either recommendation.

Clinical Picture

The patient came to my office approximately eight weeks after the initial onset of pain and swelling. ROM of all joints of the right shoulder were essentially WNL, but the patient reported that the forearm pain was reproduced passively with full shoulder flexion with elbow extension and 20° of wrist extension. Increased pain was reported with skin traction applied during the passive movements mentioned above. There were palpable "cords" along the anteromedial cubital fossa into the proximal forearm. All contractile testing of all joints of the right upper extremity was strong and painfree. MMT was generally G+ throughout and painfree to resistance. Edema was mild with the veins and tendons no longer visible at the ventral wrist. Edema extended into mid-forearm.

Treatment

1. *Gentle* moist heat to the right outstretched arm.
2. Manual stretching, including skin traction of the right shoulder complex into flexion and abduction. Performed with elbow extended with wrist extended as tolerated.
3. *Modified* manual lymphatic therapy to the right upper extremity.
4. Compression pump (Lympha Press®) × 45 minutes (added for treatments 2 and 3 only).
5. Bandaging of the right forearm/hand only.
6. Flexibility program, PREs using 2#s, variable isotonics for the upper extremity.
7. Home program of wrapping and exercise only. Slept with wrap on first two weeks only.

Outcome

Patient seen for a total of five treatments over a 4-week period of time. At time of discharge, patient was painfree with all active and passive movements of the right upper extremity. No palpable cords evident with skin traction. Edema resolved. Patient's home program consisted of daily exercise with or without the wrap (patient to decide).

Author Linda Miller, PT, Breast Cancer Physical Therapy Center, Ltd. Philadelphia, PA.

Case study reprinted with permission from *Rehabilitation Oncology* 1998;16(3):12.

References

1. Augustine, E. 1998. Historical review of external compression for lymphedema management summary of presentation at CSM. *Rehabilitation Oncology* 16(2):17–20.

2. Brennan, M. J. and Miller, L. T. 1998. Overview of treatment options and review of the current role and use of compression garments, intermittent pumps and exercise in the management of lymphedema. *Cancer* 83:2821–27.

3. Brennan, M. J. 1992. Lymphedema following the surgical treatment of breast cancer: A review of pathophysiology and treatment. *J Pain Symp Manage.* 7(2):110–16.

4. Brennan, M. J., Depompolo, R. W., Garden, F. H. 1996. Focused review: Postmastectomy lymphedema. *Arch Phys Med Rehabil.* 77: S74–80.

5. Klein, M. J., Alexander, M. A., Wright, J. M., Redmond, C. K., LaGasse, A. A. 1998. Treatment of adult lower extremity lymphedema with the Wright Linear pump: Statistical analysis of a clinical trial. *Arch PM&R* 69:202–6.

6. Zanolla, R., Monzeglio, C., Balzarini, A., Martino, G. 1984. Evaluation of the results of three different methods of postmastectomy treatment. *J Surg Oncol.* 26(3):210–13.

7. Lerner, R. 1998. What's new in lymphedema therapy in America? *International Journal of Angiology* 7:191–96.

8. Foldi, M. 1994. Treatment of lymphedema. (editorial) *Lymphology* 27:1–5.

9. Ko, D., Lerner, R., Klose, G., Cosimi, A. B. 1998. Effective treatment of lymphedema of the extremities. *Arch Surg.* 133:452–58.

10. Petrek, J. A., Pressman, P. I., Smith, R. A. 2000. Lymphedema: Current issues in research and management. *CA Cancer J Clin.* 50:292–307.

11. Dini, D., Del Mastro, L., Gozza, A., Lionetto, R., et al. 1998. The role of pneumatic compression in the treatment of postmastectomy lymphedema. A randomized phase III study. *Annals of Oncology* 9:187–90.

12. Johansson, K., Lie, E., Ekdahl, C., Tindfeldt, J. 1998. A randomized study comparing manual lymph drainage with sequential compression for treatment of postoperative arm lymphedema. *Lymphology* 31:56–64.

13. Richmand, D. M., O'Donnell, T. F., Zelikovski, A. 1985. Sequential pneumatic compression for lymphedema: A controlled trial. *Arch Surg.* 120:1116–19.

14. Pappas, C. J., O'Donnel, T. F. 1992. Long-term results of compression treatment for lymphedema. *J Vasc Surg.* 16:555–64.

15. Casley-Smith, F. R., Casley-Smith, J. R., Lasinski, B., Boris, M. 1996. The dangers of pumps in lymphoedema therapy. *Lymphology* 29:(Supplement)232–34.

16. Mortimer, P. S., et al. 1990. The measurement of skin lymph flow by isotope clearance-reliability, reproducibility, injection dynamics, and the effect of massage. *J Invest Dermatol.* 95(6):677–82.

17. Hwang, J. H., et al. 1999. Changes in lymphatic function after complex physical therapy for lympedema. *Lymphology* 32:15–21.

18. Sabris, S., Roberts, V., Cotton, L. T. 1971. Prevention of early postoperative deep vein thrombosis by intermittent compression of the leg during surgery. *Br Med J.* 4:394–96.

19. Hills, N. H., Pflug, J. J., Jeyasingh, K., et al. 1972. Prevention of deep vein thrombosis by intermittent pneumatic compression of calf. *Br Med J.* 1:131–35.

20. Sigel, B., Edelstein, A., Savitch, L., et al. 1975. Types of compression for reducing venous stasis. *Arch Surg.* 110:171–75.

21. Holford, C. P. 1976. Graded compression for preventing deep venous thrombosis. *Br Med J.* 2:969–70.

22. Lee, B. Y., Trainor, F. S., Kavner, D., et al. 1976. Noninvasive prevention of thrombosis

of deep veins of the thigh using intermittent pneumatic compression. *Surg Gyn & Obst.* 142:705–14.

23. Raines, J. K., O'Donnell, T. F., Kalisher, L., Darling, R. C. 1977. Selection of patients with lymphedema for compression therapy. *Am J Surg.* 133:430–37.

24. Casley-Smith, J. R. 1983. Varying total tissue pressures and the concentration of initial lymphatic lymph. *Microvascular Research* 25:369–79.

25. Eliska, O. and Eliskova, M. 1995. Are peripheral lymphatics damaged by high pressure manual massage? *Lymphology* 28:21–30.

26. Miller, G. E. and Seale, J. 1981. Lymphatic clearance during compressive loading. *Lymphology* 14:161–66.

27. Casley-Smith, J. R. and Bjorlin, M. O. 1985. Some parameters affecting the removal of oedema by massage-mechanical or manual. *Progress in Lymphology* 10:182–84.

28. Elhay, S. and Casley-Smith, J. R. 1976. Mathematical model of the initial lymphatics. *Microvasc Res.* 12:121–40.

29. Progress in lymphology-XIV. *Proceedings of the 14th International Congress of Lymphology.* 1993. Witte, M. H. and Witte, C. L. (eds.), The International Society of Lymphology, Zürich, Switzerland and Tucson, Arizona, USA. *Lymphology* 1994;27(Supplement):1–893.

30. Jacobs, L. F., Kepics, J., Konecne, S., et al. 1996. Lymphedema: An "orphan" disease. *PT Magazine* June, 54–61.

31. Boris, M., Weindorf, S., Lasinski, B. B. 1998. The risk of genital edema after external pump compression for lower limb lymphedema. *Lymphology* 31(1):15–20.

32. Rockson, S. G. et al. 1998. Workgroup III: Diagnosis and management of lymphedema. *Cancer* (Supplement) 83(12):2882–85.

33. Badger, C. M., Peacock, J. L., Mortimer, P. S. 2000. A randomized, controlled, parallel-group clinical trial comparing multilayer bandaging followed by hosiery versus hosiery alone in the treatment of patients with lymphedema of the limb. *Cancer* 88(12):2832–37.

34. Ryan, T. 1998. The skin and its response to movement. *Lymphology* 31:128–29.

35. Coopee, R. 2000. Use of Kinesio taping method in treatment of lymphedema. Kinesio Taping Association, Tokyo, Japan. 64–69.

36. Kase, K. 1994. Ken'l Kai Information. Tokyo, Japan. p 6.

37. Savage, R. C. 1984. The surgical management of lymphedema. *Surg Gynecol Obstet.* 160:283–90.

38. Brorson, H. and Svensson, H. 1998. Liposuction combined with controlled compression therapy reduces arm lymphedema more effectively than controlled compression therapy alone. *Plast Reconstr Surg.* 102:1058–67.

39. Miller, T. A. 1984. Surgical approach to lymphedema of the arm after mastectomy. *Am J Surg.* 148(1):152–56.

40. O'Brien, B. M., Khazanchi, R. K., Kumar, P.A.V., Dvir, E., Pederson, W. C. 1989. Liposuction in the treatment of lymphoedema: A preliminary report. *Br J Plast Surg.* 42:530–33.

41. Brorson, H. and Svensson, H. 1997. Complete reduction of lymphedema of the arm by liposuction after breast cancer. *Scand J Plast Reconstr Surg.* 31:137–43.

42. Campisi, C., Boccardo, F., Tacchella, M. 1995. Reconstructive microsurgery of lymph vessels: The personal method of lymphatic-venous-lymphatic (LVL) interpositioned grafted shunt. *Microsurgery* 16(3):161–66.

43. Piller, N. B. 1980. Lymphoedema, macrophages and benzopyrones. *Lymphology* 13:109–19.

44. Casley-Smith, J. R., Morgan, R. G., Piller, N. B. 1993. Treatment of lymphedema of the arms and legs with 5,6-benzo-alpha-pyrone. *New Engl J Med.* 1158–63.

45. Casley-Smith, J. R., Casley-Smith, J. R. 1996. Treatment of lymphedema by complex physical therapy, with and without oral and topical benzopyrones: What should therapists and patients expect. *Lymphology* 29:76–82.

46. Burgos, A., Alcaide, A., Alcoba, C., et al. 1999. Comparative study of the clincial efficacy of two different coumarin dosages in the management of arm lymphedema after treatment for breast cancer. *Lymphology* 32:3–10.

47. Loprinzi, C. L., Kugler, J. W., Sloan, J. A., et al. 1999. Lack of effect of coumarin in women with lymphedema after treatment for breast cancer. *N Engl J Med.* 340:346–50.
48. Földi, M. 1994. Treatment of lymphedema (Editorial). *Lymphology* 27:1–5.
49. Tiedjen, K. U. and Kluken, N. 1981. Isotope lymphographic research in connection with postthrombotic and lymphatic oedema under therapy with diuretics. *Progress in Lymphology* 282–85.
50. Foldi, E., Foldi, M., Clodius, L. 1989. The lymphedema chaos: A lancet. *Ann Plast Surg.* 22:505–15.
51. Casley-Smith, J. R. and Casley-Smith, J. R. 1992. Modern treatment of lymphoedema. Complex physical therapy: The first 200 Australian limbs. *J Dermatol.* 33:61–68.

PART III

MANAGEMENT ISSUES

For the health professional who is interested in treating patients with lymphedema, getting started can mean many bridges to cross and hurdles to jump. These obstacles appear in the midst of treating other patients while facing the health care challenges of today. The European model of CDT is not entirely applicable in the North American health care environment. In Europe and Australia, patients are usually seen twice a day, five days a week, until limb reduction and tissue improvement goals are met. North American medical professionals have less time to make an impact with their treatment then ever before and often run out of reimbursed visits long before interventions goals are met. Nevertheless, treating patients/clients with lymphedema is both clinically challenging and rewarding. We can expect to see more literature, expanded knowledge, and continued research in this fascinating area of human function over the next few years.

Key issues in Part III will assist the interested individual in preparing to treat this patient population while remaining on track with the financial aspects. Chapters will include: what type of education to seek, how to establish a practice which includes patients with lymphedema, documentation and reimbursement information and how to locate resource materials for patients and professionals.

6

REIMBURSEMENT ESSENTIALS
by Janice Kuperstein, PT, MSEd

"To love what you do and feel that it matters—how could anything be more fun."
KATHARINE GRAHAM
PUBLISHER, *WASHINGTON POST*

Well . . . there is the matter of getting paid for it.

INTRODUCTION

It is impossible to discuss reimbursement for lymphedema services without first reviewing a few basic concepts of reimbursement in general. This chapter is intended to put the topic in context; however, due to the complex and changing nature of health care reimbursement, it serves only as an introduction. Readers are directed to their professional associations for the most current updates.

KEY TERMINOLOGY [ADAPTED FROM *THE MANAGED HEALTH CARE DICTIONARY*]1

CPT (Current Procedural Terminology): Unique sets of five-digit codes that apply to the medical service or procedure performed by providers; established by the CPT Editorial Panel of the American Medical Association, it has become the industry coding standard for reporting.

Capitation: The provider is responsible for treating a population of patients for a prepaid payment arrangement on a per-member basis with no relationship to the amount of care actually received; a set amount of money received or paid out, based on a prepaid agreement rather than the actual cost of separate episodes of care and services delivered, usually is expressed in units of per-member-per-month (PMPM).

Carve out: Within a capitation environment, this is a type of service not included as an agreed service to be provided within the contract, therefore carved out within the PMPM or pricing structure. Carve outs may also be seen in other payment mechanisms for specialized services, which are covered under a separate payment methodology.

Case manager: A health care professional who works with patients, providers, and payers to coordinate all services deemed necessary to provide the patient with a plan of medically necessary and appropriate care. Although in most cases this is a nurse or social worker, occupational and physical therapists are increasingly entering this field.

Copayment: A payment sharing arrangement between the payer and the patient, which requires that the patient pay a specific amount per visit or a stated percentage of the bill. This is paid directly to the provider upon service.

Credentialing: The review process leading to the ultimate granting of privileges to a provider by a hospital or payer; a careful review of documents, professional license, relevant certifications, evidence of malpractice insurance, any history involving actual or alleged malpractice, and educational background of professional provider.

DRG (Diagnosis Related Groups): A system of classification for inpatient hospital services based on factors including principal diagnosis, secondary diagnosis, surgical procedures, and presence of complications; this system is used as a financing mechanism to reimburse hospitals for services rendered. The payment is based on the DRG rather than on specific services rendered.

Deductible: The minimum threshold payment that must be made by the enrollee each year before the payer begins to make payments on a shared or total basis.

Disease management: An approach to treating the entirety of a disease across the continuum of care. A focus is placed on a development of a system of care for individuals with selected diseases, to improve outcomes and reduce costs.

Fee for service: A reimbursement system in which each fee is directly associated with a service.

Fee schedule: Under a fee for service or discounted fee for service arrangement, the fee schedule is the document that outlines predetermined payments paid on given units of service. Fee schedules are often based on CPT codes.

HMO (Health Maintenance Organization): The common name given to a form of managed care involving a prepaid premium for an agreed upon set of basic and supplemental health maintenance and treatment services. Care is generally coordinated through a primary care provider. The entity must have an organized system for providing health care or ensuring health care delivery in a geographic area, and a voluntarily enrolled group of patients.

Medically necessary: The test of whether health care treatment is warranted, judged against consistency between the diagnosis, medical documentation, and the likelihood that peers within the medical community accept the treatment as necessary for the patient.

Out-of-pocket: The cost of health treatment or services that must be paid by the patient or client; these include copayment and deductible amounts as well as payment for services that are not considered covered services by the payer.

PCP (Primary Care Provider): A provider, generally a physician, who is responsible for the general health care of an individual. In many HMOs, the PCP serves in a "gatekeeper" role, requiring all covered medical care or service to be ordered by or approved by this individual for coverage under the plan.

PPO (Preferred Provider Organization): A type of managed care plan in which a group of providers agree to provide services to members under a rate or payment mechanism negotiated by the health plan.

PPS (Prospective Payment System): As established by Title VI of the Social Security Amendments of 1983, systems developed and implemented by the Health Care Financing Administration to pay for health care for Medicare patients. There are various forms of PPS in the different treatment environments, which replace the retrospective cost-based method that was initially utililized.

Participating provider: An individual provider, facility, or system agreeing to provide care or services to enrolled members of a particular health plan, according to established rates and conditions.

Payer: An organization that is engaged in providing, paying for, or reimbursing all or part of the cost of health benefits under various forms of agreements and contracts in consideration of premiums or other periodic charges; an insurer that underwrites policies and administers claims.

Per case: A reimbursement mechanism based on a fixed rate per episode of care. Rates are based on an assumed average length and intensity of intervention, and may be the same for any diagnosis, or may be negotiated for specific categories or diagnoses.

Per diem: A reimbursement mechanism in which the provider is paid an established or negotiated rate per day, rather than reimbursement for individual services rendered.

Per visit: Similar to per diem, in this reimbursement mechanism, the provider is paid for each visit the patient or client is seen, regardless of the extent of services provided.

Provider: The generic term used to describe an individual, including physicians, pharmacists, dentists, therapists, and other individuals, as well as facilities that provide health care services. Within the context of this chapter, the term will be used to denote the occupational or physical therapist. For purposes of reimbursement, other providers such as licensed massage therapists and registered nurses should consult their professional associations.

Provider profiling: The collection of provider utilization information used to assess provider practice behavior, which may include cost of treatment, duration of treatment, outcomes, and patient or client satisfaction issues.

WHO PAYS FOR HEALTH CARE?

Health care is financed through commercial insurance, which may be employer-based or private; through government financing including Medicare, Medicaid, and the military; through private out-of-pocket payments; and through Workers' Compensation. There is also a portion of health care that goes uncompensated, and is written off as charity or pro bono care.[2]

Percent of US Population Covered by Various Plans
Note that coverage is not mutually exclusive – individuals may be covered by
more than one type of health insurance during a given year

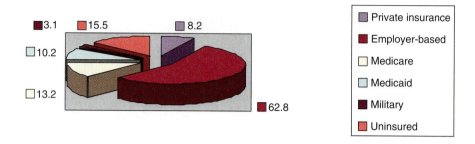

Data from U.S. Census Bureau, Current Population Survey, March 2000.[3]

COVERAGE FOR TREATMENT OF LYMPHEDEMA

Insurance coverage for the treatment of lymphedema is problematic despite advocacy by patients and providers. Coverage varies among and within payers, based on site or sites of involvement and/or based on underlying cause. This is at least partially related to the "lack of genuine understanding about lymphedema within the American medical profession in general, including those physicians who are responsible for setting coverage policy for health plans."[4] It is also due to the lack of a strong scientific base of evidence to support the efficacy of treatment. Such evidence should be accumulated as more providers collect and disseminate data and participate in clinical research protocols.

Recent improvements have been seen in coverage for lymphedema following mastectomy because of the Women's Health and Cancer Rights Act of 1998. This law amended the Employee Retirement Income Security Act of 1974 [ERISA] and subpart 3 of part B of Title XXVII of the Public Health Service Act. It requires insurers offering individual health insurance coverage, as well as all group health plans that provide medical and surgical benefits with respect to mastectomy, to provide coverage for:

- reconstruction of the breast on which the mastectomy was performed
- surgery and reconstruction of the other breast to produce a symmetrical appearance
- prostheses and physical complications for all stages of mastectomy, including lymphedema, in a manner determined in consultation with the attending physician and the patient.

Such coverage may be subject to annual deductibles and coinsurance provisions as may be deemed appropriate and as are consistent with those established for other benefits under the plan or coverage.[5]

Although the specific statute seems to indicate that such coverage is available only to individuals who elect reconstruction, the regulations, which are currently being written to more fully describe the intent of the statute, will clarify that reconstruction is not a requirement. Whether or not reconstruction is considered, this Act requires coverage for the treatment of lymphedema, and that is reportedly the way it is already being interpreted by major payers throughout the country.[6] Legislation currently being developed and introduced to Congress to address the treatment of prostate cancer and other forms of cancer is likely to include similar language to mandate coverage of complications, including lymphedema. What is *not* included in these statutes or the regulations is the type of treatment that must be provided as a covered service. Such decisions are left to the payers to determine.

Since commercial carriers are regulated at the state level, there is also wide variation in coverage for the treatment of lymphedema, other than for patients for whom there is a federal requirement, among states. Some states require health plans offered in their jurisdictions to cover such treatment, and some do not.[7] It is incumbent upon professionals to join with patients, professional associations, and other interested parties to advocate for mandated coverage in states where coverage is denied.

CPT CODES: A COMMON LANGUAGE FOR BILLING

Current Procedural Terminology [CPT] is a uniform coding system that is maintained by the AMA to provide accurate descriptive terms and uniform language in reporting medical procedures and services. The AMA supports the use of CPT by all third-party payers and urges them to implement yearly changes to CPT on a timely basis.[8] Clinicians should be aware that although the codes are consistent, the interpretation by various payers—including different carriers and fiscal intermediaries within the Medicare system—may vary.

Codes Commonly Used in Billing for Lymphedema Services

For the initial examination and evaluation, the code would depend on the professional performing the service. The appropriate codes based on discipline are:

97001—Physical therapy evaluation
97003—Occupational therapy evaluation

Neither of these two codes is time based, which means the clinician charges one unit for the complete examination/evaluation. This code should only be charged one time for the entire episode of treatment.

For re-evaluations related to a significant change in patient status, or as required monthly by some payers, the re-evaluation codes should be utilized. Again, these are based on the professional providing the service and are not timed codes.

97002—Physical therapy re-evaluation
97004—Occupational therapy re-evaluation

The use of these re-evaluation codes should be judicious. It is not appropriate to bill for a re-evaluation for weekly measurements, or for any other re-assessments that are a routine component of care.

It is important to be aware of whether payers will pay for treatment on the same day as an evaluation or re-evaluation is billed. In the case of Medicare, there is a coding edit that necessitates a modifier be utilized to indicate that the services were discrete units of service when re-evaluation is billed along with some of the other codes. Other payers may simply deny payment of any services done in conjunction with an evaluation. Such restrictions are part of the contract between the payer and provider and should be clearly communicated to all therapists impacted by that contract.

The other codes listed are not discipline-specific, so may be utilized by either professional performing the service. When billing Medicare and some other payers, a modifier is required to all codes indicating which professional is providing the service; however, there are no restrictions as long as the service is within the provider's scope of practice. When billing Medicare for any of the timed codes, the provider must be certain to follow the HCFA guidelines regarding requirements for a unit of service. This information may be found in HCFA Transmittal No. AB-00–14.60.[9] Other payers may have their own stipulations about timed codes and modifiers, which should be clearly expressed in the provider contract.

> 97140—Manual therapy techniques (e.g., Mobilization/manipulation, manual lymphatic drainage, manual traction), one or more regions, each 15 minutes: This is a timed code and may be billed in 15-minute increments. Since it explicitly includes manual lymphatic drainage in the detailed descriptor, it is obviously the code of choice for this procedure. It may also be appropriate to include the time for therapeutic bandaging under this code, charging the number of units based on time performing both portions of the treatment. Although there is a massage code [97124], which may have been used in the past, that code is not descriptive of the treatment and is no longer appropriate.[10]
>
> 97110—Therapeutic procedure, one or more areas, each 15 minutes; therapeutic exercises to develop strength and endurance, range of motion and flexibility: This code may be used for home exercise and self-manual drainage instruction. Note that codes for exercise should be selected based on the specific goal or goals of the intervention.
>
> 97112—Neuromuscular re-education of movement, balance, coordination, kinesthetic sense, posture and proprioception, each 15 minutes. Note that there are times this would be the more appropriate code based on the intent of the therapeutic procedure—again linked to the specific goal or goals.
>
> 97150—Therapeutic procedure(s), group (two or more individuals): This code should be utilized any time your intervention involves providing skilled care to two or more patients at the same time—for example, if you are teaching compression bandaging or exercise in a small group class. By definition, it does not require one-to-one patient contact by the therapist. This is not a timed code so may only be billed one time per visit. In addition, there are several different codes that are considered bundled with the group code, so you must be careful to document when the group session is discrete and separate from other services offered that day, and use the appropriate numerical modifier to indicate that in billing.
>
> 97530—Therapeutic activities, direct (one-on-one) patient contact by the provider (use of dynamic activities to improve functional performance) each 15 minutes: Some clinics use this code for lifestyle/precautions and self-bandaging instruction, and find that their payers consider this to be the preferred code for this purpose. However, the next code [97535] is

more descriptive of the intervention and has been used successfully by other clinics.

97535—Self-care/home management training (e.g., activities of daily living and compensatory training, meal preparation, safety procedures, and instructions in use of adaptive equipment), direct one-on-one contact by provider, each 15 minutes: This code is appropriate when treatment includes safety and self-care instructions for independent management, adaptive equipment use, energy conservation, work simplification, and joint protection. Lifestyle/precautions and self-bandaging instruction clearly fall into the code description and this is the code preferred by many payers.

97504—Orthotics fitting and training, upper and/or lower extremities, each 15 minutes: This code may be used for custom garment measurement. Some clinicians also use it for instruction in self-bandaging.

97016—Vasopneumatic device: Used for patients utilizing a pump in the clinic. This is not a timed code and may be billed only once per treatment session.

97703—Checkout for orthotic/prosthetic use, established patient, each 15 minutes: This code may be utilized for checking the fit of a custom garment and instructing the patient on appropriate use, care, and precautions.

Code for treatment of any of the comorbid conditions such as strength or range of motion deficits, adhesive capsulitis, postural deficits, neurological involvement, impingement syndrome, or ADL deficits is based on the specific treatments employed.[11] As with any other billing, the clinician should select codes accurately, based on the specific goals, and be certain that documentation is reflective of treatment and therefore supports the code selection.

97124—Massage, including effluerage, petrissage, and/or tapotement (stroking, compression, percussion): As noted before, this code continues to appear in the CPT manual and on some fee schedules; however, it is considerably less descriptive of the techniques involved in lymphedema management. Use the more appropriate code, 97140, unless specifically indicated otherwise by a given payer.

REIMBURSEMENT FOR SERVICES BY PRACTICE SETTING AND INSURANCE TYPE

Reimbursement for services varies by practice setting and insurance type, and may also vary by provider. The following information is based on reimbursement for occupational and physical therapists, and the licensed or certified occupational therapy or physical therapist assistants who work under their direction. Licensed massage therapists and nurses who are educated in lymphedema management are advised to consult with individual payers to determine their reimbursement policies for these professionals.

OUTPATIENT SERVICES

Since lymphedema is a chronic condition, requiring lifelong management, intervention is typically obtained as an outpatient. Outpatient services may be offered in a free-standing outpatient clinic, in a hospital-based or other facility-based outpatient department, in a comprehensive outpatient rehabilitation facility, or in some cases in a patient/client's home.

MEDICARE

The Centers for Medicare and Medicaid Services (CMS), formerly known as the Health Care Financing Administration (HCFA), administers Medicare through a network of fiscal intermediaries and carriers. Therefore, although Medicare is a federal program, there has been regional variation in how the regulations are implemented. This should be corrected under a new initiative by Medicare to standardize the interpretation and implementation of regulations through the Department of Program Integrity, however providers are advised to consult their fiscal intermediary or carrier to understand any local coverage policies.

Medicare reimburses outpatient services from Part B funds. Eligible patients will be covered for care only if it is provided according to Medicare guidelines. These require that the service be certified as medically necessary by the referring physician, be provided under a plan of care approved by the physician, and be recertified every 30 days. For specific requirements for outpatient services under Medicare, the reader is directed to the *Outpatient Provider Manual* and the Conditions of Participation. These are available in hard copy from the CMS, on their web site at *www.hcfa.gov,* or through PTManager, the Rehabilitation Leadership and Management Electronic Community, at *www.PTManager.com.*

Under Part B, Medicare pays 80% of the fee noted in a fee schedule, and the patient retains responsibility for the remaining 20% in the form of a copayment. In many cases, patients have purchased a Medicare supplement policy to cover copayments such as these.

CMS determines the payment for each CPT code based on its determination of the amount of resources consumed in providing the care or service. A system called the Resource-Based Relative Value System (RBRVS) establishes the fees based on clinical work, practice expense, and malpractice expense. This nationally uniform relative value is then multiplied by a geographical adjustment factor and a nationally uniform conversion factor, determined annually by CMS, to establish the fee schedule. An explanation of this process, sample calculations, and fee schedules are available in the Medicare Fee Schedule Calculator available as a free download on PTManager.com.

When billing patients under Medicare, the provider must also consider the implications of the Correct Coding Initiative (CCI). Implemented in 1996, the CCI is a national Medicare policy involving coding edits that restrict certain coding combinations. A code pair edit is a combination of two CPT codes that cannot be billed together because either the code pair represents services that are considered mutually exclusive, or one code is considered a component of a more comprehensive code. If the prohibited code combination is reported for the same day, only one code will be reimbursed.[12] Some, but not all, of these code combinations may be paid if a modifier is attached to the code to indicate that they were specific and distinct units of service. In these cases, the documentation should clearly reflect the distinct nature of the services provided. The codes used in lymphedema management, which are currently problematic, have been identified in the CPT descriptions previously [i.e., 97002, 97004, 97150]; however, it is important to note that edits are subject to revision by CMS on a quarterly basis. The AOTA and APTA have expressed concern about the inappropriateness of the CCI edits, and continue to work through CMS in an effort to have them removed. Meanwhile, therapists should remain current on this topic by accessing information from their professional associations, from CMS, or from the carriers or fiscal intermediaries who administer Medicare services for their clinics. The Medicare Fee Schedule Calculator from PTManager.com also includes the CCI edits and indicates those for which a modifier may be appropriate.

OTHER PAYERS

Insurance is regulated at the state level, as are Medicaid and Workers' Compensation. Therefore, there is wide variation in how these other payers reimburse providers in the outpatient environment. There may be a patient copay required under any of these payment methodologies, which must be collected by the provider. Each individual provider may be required to go through the credentialing review process before being authorized to receive payment for services. Some policies have specific requirements as to referral requirements. Under each of the mechanisms discussed, the provider should refer to the specifics of the provider contract to learn about the requirements.

Fee-for-service:
Under this payment method, the provider bills for services rendered using a fee schedule, usually based on CPT codes. The payments may be from the CMS fee schedule or any other contractually agreed-upon rate. Whether rules similar to those for Medicare are followed depends on the individual provider contract. Generally, the patient is responsible for a copay based on a percent of the charges billed.

Per visit:
Often, per visit reimbursement rates are negotiated based upon typical therapy services that are less time and labor intensive than lymphedema management. Accordingly, the per visit rate may not cover the actual cost of delivering this specialized care. When this service is a small part of a professional practice, such infrequent losses may be absorbed without consequence; however, the financial implications could be devastating to a practice that adds a large volume of patients with lymphedema without considering the financial implications. Many contracts will allow for specialized services to be "carved out" and paid under a separate methodology, and this should certainly be considered for lymphedema services.

Per case or per episode:
Although this reimbursement mechanism may involve some of the same problems noted in the per visit methodology, if there is a fairly generic case rate, it may be an excellent reimbursement methodology if the provider and payer negotiate a case rate specific for lymphedema management. Such a rate would account for the extra cost involved in the intensive treatment.

Capitation:
Under this payment methodology, the provider is paid a certain predetermined amount per member per month to provide all therapy services required by the given population. This methodology involves the greatest risk to the provider, and it is advisable that lymphedema services be negotiated as a carve out from the capitation agreement.

General Payer Issues
Preauthorization for the treatment of lymphedema is required by many commercial carriers, and is strongly recommended even when not required. The provider should

obtain information about the patient's eligibility for services and any specific limits of benefit. These limitations may involve the number of allowed visits, frequency of treatments, duration of treatment, or some other combination of restrictions. During this prior authorization procedure, the provider should also determine whether supplies would be covered by the payer and the requirements for coverage of compression garments. In this way, the patient can be prepared for any expenses that will be out of pocket, and can be an active participant in the development of an acceptable treatment plan. This preauthorization process also may serve as the beginning of an educational process for the payer regarding the benefits of the intervention.

According to the *Practice Guidelines of the American Occupational Therapy Association* and the *American Physical Therapy Association Guide to Physical Therapist Practice,* treatment planning must be based on clinical judgment, not on reimbursement issues, and patients must be apprised of any known limitations to coverage. That said, the treatment plan must also be established in collaboration with the patient, who may realistically need to consider out-of-pocket expense, as well as time and other commitments during this collaboration. It has been the experience of providers throughout the country that payers are resistant to approving daily treatment for the recommended number of weeks. They are less reluctant to approve treatment three times per week for four to six weeks. In this case, the therapist has the responsibility to consider the options with the patient and a treatment plan should be developed collaboratively.

There are several scenarios possible. In consideration of the clinical picture, the patient's knowledge and abilities regarding the home program, and the financial implications of the plan, the patient, therapist, and referral physician, if any, may determine that the payer's approval is adequate. No further action would be indicated and treatment would proceed according to the approved plan of care. Alternatively, the overall picture may suggest that the frequency and/or duration of therapy approved by the payer would be inadequate. In such a case, the therapist should assist in an appeal of the payer's position by documenting a thorough clinical justification. The patient should decide whether to proceed with the more intensive plan with the knowledge that there may be additional out-of-pocket expenses, or to elect the less intensive plan while awaiting a decision from the payer. If the plan is altered for financial considerations, documentation should clearly reflect that this was the patient's decision following a full discussion of risks, benefits, and alternatives.

Assuming the health plan denies approval for the recommended clinical treatment, the therapist should advise the patient of her or his right to appeal health plan decisions. The Member Services Department, which can usually be reached through a toll-free number on the back of the enrollment card, will provide information about the process for appeals.[13]

When working with commercial insurance companies, it is helpful to provide information about the efficacy of treatment, as well as the intensity of service. Educate the payer about the long-term effects of lymphedema and that the emphasis of your planned intervention program is long-term self-management and prevention. It is also helpful to educate the payer regarding the possible need for a repeat course of therapy in the future. Finally, involving the payer's case manager in discussing coverage issues may expedite the review process and enhance likelihood of optimal coverage.

A difficult dilemma for patients and providers of lymphedema services occurs when the approved therapy providers for a given HMO or PPO are unaware of the current treatment approach to lymphedema management and utilize the more traditional, and generally less effective, modalities. When provided with appropriate references, patients have been successful in obtaining payment for out-of-network providers from various commercial carriers; however, in many cases such approval is obtained only after a failed course of treatment from the participating provider. This reinforces the critical need for scientifically sound studies assessing clinical outcomes—functional abilities, quality of life, and overall cost of care—and should become a focus of advocacy by patients and providers.

Disease Management:

As more payers are implementing a disease management approach to high risk, high volume, and/or expensive disorders, lymphedema management should be one they consider. A therapy practice with expertise in this area should approach payers with which they have an existing contract, as well as those who contract only with other providers, to offer a comprehensive management program at a negotiated price. This may be at a fee for service, per diem, or case, rate based on contract negotiations. The provider should be prepared to provide literature on the efficacy of treatment with a focus on long-term prevention, evidence of specialized training including certification, and data on your individual practice experience. Demonstration of outcome studies to include volume reduction, prevention of complications, patient satisfaction, and improved quality of life would provide added incentive for a health plan to contract with you for this specialized service. Such information is also valuable as providers see the initiation of provider profiling by various payers. The payers should be presented with the outcome information to supplement their own data on cost of care.

Supplies:

Clinics have had varying success in obtaining reimbursement for the bandaging supplies. Although Medicare does not generally cover supplies, many of the commercial carriers do cover them. This is something that should be discovered during the preauthorization process so the patient can be notified in advance. When supplies are not covered by the payer, the patient may be billed for them separately, or may be directed to purchase them at a local vendor prior to treatment.

Compression Garments:

Again coverage varies by payer, and sometimes even by time or method of request from the same payer. Most commercial carriers will cover garments as long as the documentation clearly indicates the need for a custom compression garment; however, they are unlikely to pay for a sufficient number of garments. Considering the typical recommendation that the patient have two garments to allow for cleaning and alternate-day wear and should replace garments based on wear up to several times per year, patients often must still pay for at least part of the cost out of pocket.

Although Medicare typically does not cover garments at all, there have been reports of patients who have appealed several times—for one patient all the way to an administrative law judge—and have received payment on an individual basis.[14] This suggests that patients, with the assistance of providers, should be persistent in appealing denials of any reasonable claims.

PRIVATE PAY

Clients/patients may choose to pay for lymphedema treatment independently in cases in which their insurance coverage doesn't cover these services, coverage is limited, or their chosen provider is not a participating provider for their payer. It is important to recognize that patients have this right, and therapists should not feel uncomfortable charging a fair rate to cover all costs as well as a reasonable profit. It may be easier to accept when we consider how many people pay out of pocket for complementary and alternative treatments, or personal training, based on their own desire to obtain these services. Some providers may simply choose to not accept insurance payment given the complexity and variation in contracts, and may instead require patients to pay out of pocket and bill the insurance company themselves.

These patients should be treated in the same way as others, with treatment decisions made based on clinical judgments and collaboration with the individual. Documentation standards should be maintained whether or not the person intends to file bills with an insurance company, in compliance with professional standards and licensure requirements.

INPATIENT SERVICES

Although, as noted, most lymphedema management is provided on an outpatient basis, there are instances in which treatment is initiated, or even completed, in various inpatient environments.

ACUTE CARE HOSPITALS

Patients may have their initial diagnosis of lymphedema made during an inpatient hospital stay for treatment of infection, cellulitis, or even an unrelated disorder. In these cases, lymphedema management would appropriately be initiated as soon as the medical condition is stable enough to allow intervention. Given the short average length of stay, it is also appropriate to initiate planning for outpatient follow-up during this initial intervention.

Medicare:
Acute care hospitals are reimbursed for inpatient stays for Medicare recipients based on the DRG system of prospective payment. As noted previously, this is a system of classification based on factors including principal diagnosis, secondary diagnosis, surgical procedures, and presence of complications. The hospital is reimbursed based on the DRG designation, not on specific services rendered. If lymphedema management is initiated during the hospital stay, all services and supplies are included, with no additional expense to the patient. This is an appropriate course of action when the initiation of treatment would have an impact on the acute condition. When long-standing lymphedema is diagnosed in the hospital but is unrelated to the hospital admission, it may be more appropriate to simply educate the patient on the treatment and wait to initiate care on an outpatient basis.

Other Payers:
Again, there is wide variation among payers in payment to hospitals. Under a fee-for-service arrangement, the payer would be reimbursed for the charges incurred, some-

times at a contractually negotiated discount. In most cases, these charges would be based on the individual charges billed in provision of care. Many payers negotiate per diem rates with hospitals, often based on acuity, and in these cases, all services and supplies would be included in the per diem rate.

NURSING FACILITIES

Residents of nursing facilities, who require lymphedema services, may fall into several categories in terms of reimbursement.

Medicare Part A:

Medicare Part A covers the first 100 days of treatment in a skilled nursing facility for covered beneficiaries, if they were admitted to the nursing facility within 30 days of a hospital stay of at least 3 days' duration and continue to require skilled services. The reimbursement mechanism for these patients is a form of prospective payment based on resource utilization groups (RUGS), which are determined from a comprehensive assessment tool—the Minimum Data Set (MDS)—completed for each patient. All therapy services and supplies for lymphedema management would be included in the payment based on the RUGS designation.

Other Payers:

In most cases, nursing facility residents are either paying for their residential care through private funds, through Medicaid, or in a small percentage of cases through private long-term care insurance. Under these circumstances, lymphedema treatment would be billed to the individual's health insurance carrier, whether that is Medicare, Medicaid, or some other payer, much as if the patient were receiving an outpatient procedure.

HOME HEALTH

Individuals with lymphedema who meet the criteria of being home bound as defined by their payer may require management in the home health setting. [Clinicians are advised to assure the correct height treatment surface to avoid injury to themselves when treating in a patient's home.] There are various reimbursement mechanisms based on the payer, as well as on the relationship of the therapist to the home health agency.

Medicare:

As of October 1, 2000, Medicare has implemented a prospective payment system for their beneficiaries receiving home health. Payment is based on a comprehensive assessment using the Outcomes and Assessment Information Set [OASIS], which is administered to each patient on admission to the home health agency. A payment is determined for each 60-day episode of care, which includes all services required. If a patient were to require lymphedema management in this setting, the cost of the therapist's time as well as the supplies would come out of the 60-day payment allotment. Since this new form of PPS was just recently implemented, it is unknown whether home health agencies will be reluctant to accept patients requiring the intensive therapy indicated for patients with lymphedema.

Other Payers:

Although the OASIS is administered to all patients admitted to the care of home health agencies, reimbursement for services by other payers may not be based on this assessment. Contractual negotiations between the payer and the agency would determine the reimbursement mechanism in place. Common reimbursement mechanisms include discounted fee for service or per diem.

CONCLUSION

As with any other rehabilitation services, reimbursement for lymphedema management varies based on the payer and the setting of intervention. Careful documentation addressing impairments, functional limitations, functional goals, and an accurate description of the treatment provided are essential in all environments to enhance reimbursement. Moreover, as the health care reimbursement system continues to evolve, and as patients, payers, and providers continue to advocate for coverage, more changes are likely. Clinicians would be best able to follow these emerging developments through their professional associations and through the National Lymphedema Network or other similar organizations.

References

1. Rognehaugh, R. 1998. *The Managed Health Care Dictionary,* 2nd ed. Gaithersburg, Maryland: Aspen Publishers, Inc.
2. Kristy, W. 1999. Basics of health care financing and reimbursement. In K. A. Curtis (ed.), *The Physical Therapist's Guide to Health Care.* Thorofare, NJ: SLACK Inc.
3. U.S. Census Bureau. *www.census.gov.hhes/ hlthins/hlthin99/dtable1.html*
4. Schuch, W. J. National Lymphedema Network Question Corner. *www.lymphnet.org/ question10–00.html*
5. Pub. L. No. 105–277, § 902
6. Connor, Mark. Office of Health Plan Standards. Personal communication.
7. Runowicz, C. 1998. Lymphedema after cancer. *Health News* 4(5):1–2
8. PL 70.974, Sub. Res. 809, A-92
9. HCFA Transmittal No. AB-00-14.60. Questions and answers regarding the prospective payment system (PPS) for outpatient rehabilitation services and physical medicine current procedural terminology (CPT) coding guidance. *www.hcfa.gov/ pubforms/transmit/2000/memo/comm_date_ dsc. htm*
10. Fearon, Helene M. PT, Rehabilitation Representative to the American Medical Association CPT Editorial Panel. Personal communication.
11. Carson, C. J., Coverly, B., Lasker-Hertz, S. 1999. The incidence of co-morbidities in the treatment of lymphedema. *Journal of Oncology Management* 8(4): 13–17.
12. American Physical Therapy Association. *apta.org/Advocacy/top20/Correct_Coding_ Initiative*
13. Cohn, R. 1999. The wise consumer: Making choices for your health. *PT Magazine* 7(10):14–15 *internet.apta.org/pt_magazine/ oct99/consumer.html*
14. Lasinski, B. B. National Lymphedema Network Question Corner. *www.lymphnet. org/question01–00.html*

7

ESTABLISHING A PRACTICE IN LYMPHEDEMA MANAGEMENT

"In addition to progress in research, doctors are becoming more aware of and sensitive to lymphedema, qualified lymphedema therapists are growing in numbers, lymphedema centers are proliferating, *and networks of lymphedema patients are getting together to place this long-neglected condition on the map."*
JOAN SWIRSKY, R.N., AND DIANE SACKETT NANNERY, AUTHORS

INTRODUCTION

Whether it is a corner of a current department or a free-standing clinic, many clinicians have a goal of establishing a practice that is focused on patients with lymphedema. Because of the unique nature of the treatments, the particular need for privacy, and the amount of specialized equipment and supplies, it is reasonable to hope and plan for a space dedicated specifically to the needs of this patient population.

For purposes of this text, the proposed specialty practice will be referred to as a Center. This proposed Center is to open with two health professionals specifically educated in lymphedema management. Later expansion plans could extrapolate this information to estimate needs.

Differences in regional costs will affect the expenses shown here. Existing space and equipment, which has shared use with other staff and patient/client types such as a gymnasium or reception area, will affect cost totals as well.

A LYMPHEDEMA CENTER: PROGRAM OVERVIEW

In alignment with the National Lymphedema Network, therapists at the Center provide a five-part treatment plan for lymphedema. Patient care is provided to individuals with lymphedema following but not limited to cancer surgery, burn injury, radiation therapy, chronic wound treatment, surgery, trauma, sports injury, or vascular compromise affecting the lymphatic system.

INSTITUTIONAL IMPACT

The development of a Lymphedema Center can be important to the critical success factors of an institution:

- *Customer satisfaction:* Achievement of customer loyalty by providing a private and confidential area for treatment and education.
- *Employee satisfaction:* Allows staff with specialization to maintain and enhance their knowledge and skills.
- *Customer loyalty:* Provision of the service to internal referral base, if appropriate, to allow maintenance of the customer within the system. Provision of the service to external referral base to serve the community.
- *Regional or national recognition:* This might be within the institutional focus of cancer services, since lymphedema care is used within the postoperative care of some cancer patients.

LEADERSHIP

The Center would be under the direction and leadership of an individual with specialized education in lymphedema management. There should be physician/practitioner support for the Center. When there is a nearby university, gaining support of the faculty for the Center may enhance opportunities for research collaboration. This could add to the knowledge on lymphedema and provide evidence necessary to optimize reimbursement.

MARKETING AND EDUCATION

The Center business plan would include the ability to increase the market share of patients with lymphedema through:

- National Lymphedema Network (NLN) registration that would provide customer access to the NLN website including the Center's program, staff names, and credentials. See Chapter 8 for more information about the NLN.
- Direct mailings to physician/practitioner referral base.
- Communications with physicians/practitioners within the healthcare network regarding the development of the Center and what it can provide for patients.
- Media coverage of the opening of the Center that would include phone numbers, website information, as well as an overview of the program.
- Increased public awareness of lymphedema through marketing strategies associated with Breast Cancer Awareness month, Race for the Cure, support groups, and so on.
- Development of a portable presentation board that could be used at health fairs and other health-related events.
- Development of an informational brochure for distribution to the public.
- Newsletter sent quarterly to referring practitioners with case studies, patient statistics, updates on activities of the staff related to lymphedema.
- Provider relations inservices to educate payers about available treatment options.

FINANCIAL IMPACT

SPACE

To develop and become a designated Lymphedema Center, a minimum space commitment of approximately 1650 square feet would provide a small but efficient area to pioneer the program. Expansion in staff or patient load would require additional space and equipment. Allocating space for at least two treatment rooms and two bathrooms with showers would allow patients to receive their total care with an appropriate level of privacy within the same clinic. Providing a space of this type may serve as a marketing tool in addition to serving the patient population well. This proposal would allow the following:

> *Reception Area* (1) 300 sq. ft.
>> Containing reception and therapist documentation areas; patient records storage; patient waiting area; display for patient education materials.
>
> *Treatment Rooms* (2) 200 sq. ft. (or 100 sq. ft. each)
>> Containing treatment table, lavatory, casework for storage of patient care materials (examination and treatment supplies), one chair, one rolling stool. If there are future plans for expansion, additional treatment room dimensions should be included in the total square feet estimates.
>
> *Rest Rooms* (2) 110 sq. ft. (or 55 sq. ft. each)
>> Accessible from reception area as well as treatment rooms and must include a shower within each.*
>
> *Storage Closet* (2) 40 sq. ft. (or 20 sq. ft. each)
>> Space for storage of bulk bandages, other department stock items, and audio/visual education equipment.
>
> *Gymnasium* (1) 1000 sq. ft.
>> Containing rehabilitation equipment and space for exercise mats to accommodate 10 to 20 persons. This will also serve as a group education/conference room.

Note: If you do not plan to expand your staff or patient services, and if your schedule will allow for staggering patients by 30 minutes between therapists, you might be able to function with one rest room with shower. Two rooms with showers, however, will allow the most scheduling options, greater opportunity for expansion, and the assurance that if one room is out of service there is still at least one functioning room for patients to use. If treatment includes wound care in addition to other intervention, the ability to use the shower room for wound care will keep waste products out of the treatment area and allow for easier clean-up after a wound treatment. If future expansion plans include another treatment room, they may not necessitate a third rest room with shower.

EQUIPMENT

Equipment needed should include hi-lo treatment tables (two); treatment supplies—automatic digital sphygmomanometer, tape measures, goniometers, reflex hammer, Doppler ultrasound for ABI calculation (optional); exercise equipment—treadmill, ergometer, pulley weights, free weights, therapy balls; office supplies—two computers with hardware and software, TV/VCR, AV stand, video camera, still photo camera; and furniture for reception area and treatment rooms.

The projected cost of equipment is approximately US $55,000.

SUPPLIES

The Center stock items should include *one case* of each of the different sizes of compression bandages, foam, stockinette, and so on. See information on bandages and garments in Chapters 4 and 8. Purchase of bandages and other patient supplies can be handled in a variety of ways:

- Patient goes to local vendor and purchases a set of bandages as designated by the therapist.
- Patient is given list of bandages needed and purchases them through a mail-order vendor.
- Patient purchases them from your facility. (Consider the markup formulas for your facility as they may put the price of the bandages out of reach for the patient.)
- Patient purchases bandages elsewhere but you supply the occasional replacement as needed. You may charge the patient outright or have them trade out the bandages when they have the chance to purchase replacements.
- When appropriate, you may include the cost of supplies in your charges as established by the payer.

Off-the-shelf compression garments are costly to maintain as department stock unless your Center is in an established clinic with a well-supplied stock closet. In the beginning, you may wish to establish a relationship with a few local vendors for the off-the-shelf garments. Later, as your volume increases, you may be able to stock your own garments. The majority of patients have the best adherence rate and satisfaction with custom garments. Custom garment billing is often handled differently from off-the-shelf billing. As noted in Chapter 6, some payers will pay for garments given sufficient documentation of medical necessity.

Other items, such as specialized skin care products, self-help videos, small exercise equipment, and positioning devices, should be stocked based on your available start-up funds and your markup formulas. As your volume increases you may be able to stock more of these to sell to patients. A free-standing clinic is not restricted by facility markup policies, which sometimes make supply charges prohibitive.

The projected cost of stock bandage supplies for start-up is approximately US $1,275. (The cost of other stock items will vary based on start-up funds and are not listed here.)

PERSONNEL

The Center will begin with two health professionals with specific education in lymphedema management. The heavy physical demands of the manual therapy and bandaging portions of the intervention require stamina and strength. Two professionals can assist each other, cover for each other during absence, provide physical relief and professional encouragement. If it is a free-standing clinic, the Center will need one additional staff employee to serve as receptionist, billing clerk, and therapy technician.

Personnel expenses will include salary plus benefits, including professional liability insurance, continuing education, and other options as appropriate.

OTHER EXPENSES

If adding a Lymphedema Center to an existing clinic, many of these costs will be easily identified. If starting a new free-standing Center, decisions about location and amenities will significantly influence the actual expenses incurred.

Fixed: rent, utilities, equipment, insurance
Variable: supplies, linens

COMMON CHALLENGES (TO THE SUCCESS OF YOUR CENTER)

Challenge #1: The greatest challenge to the success of a practice focusing on the treatment of lymphedema is the *lack of education and appropriate referrals* from referring practitioners. This should be easily remedied by providing information referenced throughout this text. The Lymphedema Center will allow these practitioners to offer their patients a promising treatment alternative, where before there were none. A rewarding partnership should readily be built.

Challenge #2: The second challenge will be obtaining *adequate reimbursement* from payer sources. There are three scenarios that should be considered.

First, when adding lymphedema management as a new service within an existing clinic, many of the fixed costs may be covered already. Additionally, provider contracts will already be in place. As noted in Chapter 6, providers with existing contracts should carefully review the payment methodology and rate before initiating a new program. This is to ensure that the rate will not be below the actual cost. You must negotiate contracts that allow for adequate reimbursement to cover all expenses plus profit. *Provider contracts*[1] generally include the following sections:

- *Purpose:* Defines the parties involved and states the purpose and intent of the contractual relationship.
- *Definitions:* Defines the terms utilized throughout the document.
- *Obligations:* Establishes the specific responsibilities incumbent upon each party, including such issues as administrative procedures for authorization, billing, documentation, and reimbursement.
- *Terms and termination:* Outlines the effective date and duration of the contract, as well as renewal and termination provisions.
- *Miscellaneous:* Includes provisions relating to contract amendment and security of proprietary information.

In the second scenario, the case of a new clinic, relationships with payers as well as referral sources will need development. Contracts should be carefully considered to assure financial viability. See Chapter 6 for more information.

Finally, should the provider choose to establish a program accepting only patients who privately pay for care, a reasonable charge must be determined. In all cases of developing charges/fee schedules, the clinician must consider all costs involved in providing the service. If starting a new clinic rather than adding a service to an existing clinic, appropriate state and local government agencies should be contacted regarding "new business" regulations.

Challenge #3: The third challenge relates to *patient adherence* issues. Much of the success of the intervention and long-term limb reduction depends on the willingness and ability of the patient to adhere to the treatment program both in Phase I and Phase II. Several studies are in progress to examine how to measure and influence patient adherence. Adequate patient education, patient satisfaction, and quality of life perceptions are some of the keys to improving adherence.

Challenge #4: The fourth challenge is the risk of *professional isolation*. Unless established in a large area with many specially educated professionals, staff in the Center will need to seek support for professional growth through continuing education, reading current literature, special interest groups, and networking activities. Close contact with a supportive and knowledgeable practitioner is helpful.

SUMMARY

This chapter has suggested a plan for establishing a Lymphedema Center. There are still many details to consider before the Center could accept its first patients. Many of those will be specific to a particular site and cannot be anticipated in a text of this size. When planning for a Center, it can be beneficial to refer to a text that has been specifically written to assist health professionals. One such book, which can be used by a variety of professionals, includes valuable information such as how to get paid, common facility design mistakes to avoid, and using marketing dollars wisely.[2]

References

1. Knight, W. 1998. *Managed Care.* Gaithersburg, MD: Aspen Publishers, Inc.
2. Nosse, L. F., Friberg, D. G., Kovacek, P. R. 1999. *Managerial and Supervisory Principles for Physical Therapists*, 1st ed. Baltimore, MD: Williams & Wilkins.

8
RESOURCES FOR HEALTH PROFESSIONALS

"... I gained a deeper appreciation of the degree to which literally millions of people—men, women, and children—were suffering from lymphedema and had nowhere to go and no one to turn to for information."

JOAN SWIRSKY, R.N., AUTHOR AND ADVOCACY JOURNALIST

INTRODUCTION

Listed in this chapter are sources of information on a variety of topics related to lymphedema management. Patients could also be directed to the "Resources" section of the book *Coping with Lymphedema*[1] for information and links to a variety of information relating to lymphedema. Addresses and telephone numbers are subject to change.

The following single page handout has been created for patient education opportunities. It has been written in language understandable to the general public. The information should be presented by a specially educated professional who can address the individual's specific needs and concerns as they relate to the general list. The suggestions do not require drastic life changes and could be followed by any individual seeking a healthy lifestyle.

To educate patients on how to assess the prevention and control guidelines, they should be advised to *avoid activities that can trigger a further decrease of the transport capacity of the lymph vessels and/or unnecessarily increase the lymphatic fluid and protein load of the lymphatic system in the affected region.* Michael Foldi (1998)

GUIDELINES FOR THE PREVENTION AND CONTROL OF LYMPHEDEMA

Skin Care: Avoid injuries to the skin that can lead to bacterial or fungal infection.

- Keep skin meticulously clean and moist using a gentle cleanser with a moisturizer every day.
- Keep nails and toenails cut short. Avoid manicures, pedicures, and artificial nails. Do not cut cuticles. Use a nail file to shorten nails.
- Avoid heat in general but specifically to your involved limb. Avoid hot packs, moist heat, heating pads, hot air, fireplace heat, sun, dishwashing, hot tubs or whirlpools, saunas, sunbathing, and so on.
- Avoid wounds or scratches. Wear gloves for indoor and outdoor work. Avoid insect bites and pet scratches. Use an electric razor to shave underarms and legs. Wear shoes when outdoors if a lower extremity is involved.

Exercise and activity: Exercise is an important part of staying healthy.

- If you experience discomfort in the limb at risk, elevate the limb, and cut back on your activity.
- Avoid lifting more than 15 pounds with an affected upper extremity unless specific strengthening exercises have been initiated under the supervision of a qualified professional.
- Swim, walk, or do specially prescribed exercises. Discuss all forms of exercise with your therapist.
- Talk to your therapist about exercises and activities that have been shown to increase the likelihood of the onset of lymphedema in some people. Repetitive and/or vigorous movements of the involved extremity should be carefully monitored at work or leisure.
- Avoid prolonged sitting, or any activity that will restrict lymph flow at the site of the lymph nodes especially behind the knee, in the groin, at the elbow, and in the underarm area. Try to change position frequently during daytime hours.

Extra precautions for the involved limb: Avoid external pressure, which might slow or stop lymph flow.

- Avoid tight-fitting undergarments and clothing.
- Do not sleep on your involved side.
- Do not allow your blood pressure to be taken, blood to be drawn, or an injection to be given to the involved extremity.
- Before traveling by air, consult with a qualified professional about the use of a compression garment to assist in the prevention of potential swelling.
- Avoid deep massage to the affected limb. When in doubt, ask your therapist.

Diet and Nutrition: Good nutrition leads to good health.

- There is no special diet to prevent or control lymphedema, but it is in your best interest to practice excellent nutrition habits and to maintain a normal weight. Some research has shown that obesity increases the likelihood that a person will develop lymphedema.

Problems with your involved limb: Watch for danger signs.

- Watch for signs of infection: heat, pain, redness, swelling, chills, fever. See your physician immediately. Also see your physician for rashes on the affected limb, wounds that are slow to heal, or pain in an involved extremity.
- Seek treatment for any signs or symptoms of lymphedema: numbness, tingling, tight feeling, stiffness, or swelling **anywhere** on the limb at risk. Report increases in size to your physician. Be persistent about getting follow-up care.

LYMPHEDEMA MANAGEMENT EDUCATION PROGRAMS*

There are a number of organizations in North America, Europe, and Australia that offer education in various forms of manual therapy, lymphedema bandaging, skin care, and exercise. These courses vary in length, intensity, and rationale for their particular style of manual applications. Currently the most comprehensive instruction in MLD and lymphedema bandaging is taught through courses that culminate in a certification exam. These courses will help to prepare the participant to sit for the National Certification Exam for lymphedema therapists, which is administered by the Lymphology Association of North America (LANA).

Academy of Lymphatic Studies
Office: Sebastian, FL
Phone: (800) 863–5935
Director: Joachim Zuther

The Casley-Smith School
Office: Malvern, Australia
Phone (from US): 011–61-8–8271-2198
Fax: 011–61-8–8271-8776
Director: Dr. Judith Casley-Smith

Casley-Smith Training Centers in North America:

Lymphedema Therapy Center, Inc.   and   Boris-Lasinski School
Office: Roswell, GA   Office: Woodbury, Long Island, NY
Phone: (770) 518–4700   Phone: (516) 364–2200
Director: DeCourcy Squire   Director: Dr. Marvin Boris

Coast to Coast School of Lymphedema Management LeDuc Method
Office: Temecula, CA
Phone: (909) 600–0634
Director: Anne-Marie Vaillant-Newman

The Foldi School—Privateschule Foldi GMBH
Office: Merzhausen, Germany
Phone (from US): 011–49-761–406921
Fax: 01149-761-406983
Director: Prof. Michael Foldi
Website: *www.foeldiklinik.de/engl/info.htm*

Klose Norton Training & Consulting, Inc.
Office: Red Bank, NJ
Phone: (877) 842–4414
Fax: (732) 842–5299
Director: Guenter Klose
Website: *www.klosenorton.com*

Lymph Drainage Therapy—Upledger Institute
Office: West Palm Beach, FL
Phone: (800) 311–9204 ext 92008
Director: Dr. Bruno Chikly and Renee Romero

*For a complete listing of program codes, eligibility for courses, and current address changes, go to the National Lymphedema Network website at *www.lymphnet.org*

Dr. Vodder School of North America
Office: Victoria, BC Canada
Phone: 250-598-9862
Director: Robert Harris

To locate health professionals trained by these programs, see the individual websites where graduates of the programs are often listed by state. The NLN website also lists the locations of specifically trained professionals by state.

Key contacts:

The American Cancer Society
1599 Clifton Road, NE
Atlanta, GA 30329
Phone: (800) 227-2345
Website: *www.cancer.org*

American Occupational Therapy Association
4720 Montgomery Lane
Bethesda, MD 20814
Phone: (800) 377-8555
Fax: (301) 652-7711
Website: *www.aota.org*

American Physical Therapy Association
1111 North Fairfax St.
Alexandria, VA 22314
Phone: (800) 999-2782
Fax: (703) 684-7343
Website: *www.apta.org*

British Lymphology Society (BLS)
Administration Office, Mrs. Helen Snoad
Bls Administration Center
PO Box 1059
Caterham, Surrey CR3 6ZU
England
Phone: 01883 330 253
Fax: 01883 330 254
Email: *helensnoad@blsac.demon.co.uk*
Website: *www.lymphoedema.org/bls*

(Membership open to all healthcare professionals, information on treatment research, equipment, and networking. Membership fee, newsletter, annual conference.)

International Society of Lymphology
Central Office address:
M.H. Witte MD, Sec. Gen'l, ISL,
University of Arizona—College of Medicine
Department of Surgery
PO Box 245063
1501 N. Campbell Ave
Tucson, AZ 85724-5063
Phone: (520) 626-6118
Email: *lymph@u.arizona.edu*
Website: *www.u.arizona.edu/~witte/ISL.htm*

(Founded to advance and disseminate knowledge in the field of lymphology, establish relations between researchers and clinicians, and strengthen experimental and clinical investigation. Membership fee, quarterly journal, international conference.)

Lymphology Association of North America
(LANA)
1800 NW Market Street, Ste. 203
Seattle, WA 98107-3908
Email: *lana@snonet.org*
Website: *www.snonet.org/lana*

(Administers the National Certification
Exam in North America)

National Lymphedema Network (NLN)
1611 Telegraph Avenue, Suite 1111
Oakland, CA 94612-2138
Phone: (510) 208-3200
Hotline: (800) 541-3259
Fax: (510) 208-3110
Email: *nln@lymphnet.org*
Website: *www.lymphnet.org*

(Nonprofit membership organization
that provides education to patients,
healthcare professionals, and the
public about lymphedema.
Quarterly newsletter, biannual
conference.)

National Alliance of Breast Cancer Organizations
(NABCO)
9 East 37th St, 10th Floor
New York, NY 10016
Information Services Staff phone: (888) 806-2226
Fax: (212) 689-1213
Email: *NABCOinfo@aol.com*
Website: *www.nabco.org*

(Nonprofit information and
education resource on breast
cancer and a national force in
patient advocacy in North America)

Contacts for Products:

Academy of Lymphatic Studies
10753 US Hwy #1
Sebastian, FL 32958
Phone: (800) 863-5935
Fax: (561) 589-0306

(Bandaging supplies)
(This company is owned and operated by
an experienced lymphedema therapist.)

Barton Carey
PO Box 421
Perrysburg, OH 43552
Phone: (800) 421-0444
Fax: (419) 874-0888

(Compression garments)

BSN-Jobst, Inc.
Box 471048
Charlotte, NC 28247-1048
Phone: (800) 537-1063
Fax: (800) 336-5578
Website: *www.jobst-usa.com*

(Manufacturer and distributer of Elvarex
compression garments and
BSN-Jobst bandaging supplies—see
Figures 8.2a–d)

Camp International, Inc.
744 W. Michigan Ave
PO Box 89
Jackson, MI 49204
Phone: (800) 788-2267
Fax: (517) 789-3299

(Compression garments)

CircAid
9323 Chesapeake Drive, Suite B-2
San Diego, CA 92123
Phone: (858) 576-3550
Fax: (858) 576-3555
Email: *info@circaid.com*
Website: *www.circaid.com*

(Nonelastic limb containment systems)

JUZO (Julius Zorn, Inc.)
PO Box 1088
80 Chart Road
Cuyahoga Falls, OH 44223
Phone: (800) 222-4999
Fax: (800) 645-2519

(Compression garments)

Kinesio Taping Association
11005 Spain NE, Suite 21
Albuquerque, NM 87111
Phone: (505) 797-7818
Fax: (505) 338-2170
Email: *info@kinesiotaping.com*
Website: *www.kinesiotaping.com*

(Kinesio® Tex Tape, information on courses)

Lymphedema Products, LLC
326 Broad St, 2nd Floor
Red Bank, NJ 07701
Phone toll free: (877) 842-4414
Fax: (732) 842-5299
Email: *Steve@klosenorton.com*
Website: *www.lymphedemaproducts.com*
Contact: Steve Norton

(Lymphedema bandaging supplies and other products. This company is owned and operated by experienced lymphedema therapists. Their line of products has been selected based on their benefits when used in combination with CDT.)

LogiMed
505 W. Olive Ave, Suite 330
Sunnyvale, CA 94086
Phone: (408) 732-8400
Fax: (408) 732-8830

(Tribute™ lymphedema products for a variety of body regions including the head and neck)

Lohmann & Rauscher, Inc.
P.O. Box 19165
Topeka, KS 66619-0165
Phone: (888) 265-0199
Fax: (888) 794-0199
Email: *lrmedus@smithorthopedics.com*
Website: *www.lohmann-rauscher.com*

(Manufacturer and distributer of Lohmann lymphedema bandaging supplies)

Medassist-OP, Inc.
P.O. Box 758
Palm Harbor, FL 34682
Phone: (800) 521-6664
Fax: (502) 897-2508

(Arm Assist®/Leg Assist® Nonelastic limb containment system)

Medi USA, L.P.
76 West Seegers Road
Arlington Heights, IL 60005
Phone: (800) 633-6334
Fax: (708) 640-0209

(Compression garments)

Mego Afek Medical Division
Kibbutz Afek 30042
Israel
Fax: (972)-4-878-4148
Email: *deborah@megoafek.co.il*
Website: *www.lympha-press.com*

(Lympha Press® pneumatic compression devices:
upper extremity with shoulder attachment,
overlapping pants, standard Lympha Press®,
Lympha Press mini devices)

North American Rehabilitation
PMB 85
325 S. Washington Ave
Kent, WA 98032
Phone: (800) 300-5512
Fax: (253) 630-8111

(Lymphedema bandaging supplies and other
products)

Peninsula Medical, Inc.
PO Box 66149
Scotts Valley, CA 95067-6149
Phone: (800) 293-3362
Fax: (831) 430-9068
Website: *www.noblemed.com*

(ReidSleeve® nonelastic limb containment system
and other lymphedema products)

Sigvaris, Inc.
PO Box 570
Bradford, CT 06405
Phone: (800) 322-7744
Fax: (203) 481-5488

(Compression garments)

Tri-D Corporation
800 Industry Drive
Tukwila, WA 98188
Phone: (206) 575-1656
Fax: (206) 575-9296
Toll free: (866) 888-5684
Email: *rovig@jovipak.com*
Website: *www.jovipak.com*

(JoVi Pak™, self-care videos for patients).
Lymphedema products designed by a lymphedema
therapist. See photo and description of JoVi Pak™
in this chapter.)

FIGURE 8-1 Application of the JoVi Pak™ Arm Liner

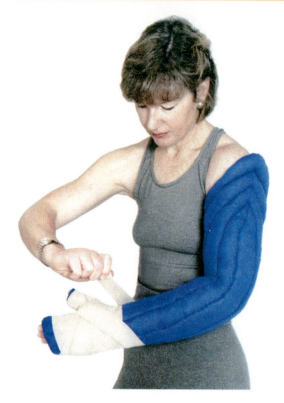

The model is demonstrating a typical application by wrapping a short-stretch bandage over the JoVi Pak™. (Courtesy of JoVi Pak, a Division of Tri-D Corporation)

Most lymphedema therapists utilize custom pieces under short-stretch bandaging to assist in softening fibrotic tissue for appropriate patients. Chipped foam under bandaging increases the efficacy of the bandaging in softening tissue where needed. The chips allow channels for lymphatic fluid to continue to move through pathways even under compression wraps. Patients often wear a chip bag under short-stretch bandaging at night. Therapists typically fabricate bags of chips utilizing leftover foam pieces and tubular bandage. Other names of items that achieve similar results are: muffs, Schneider Packs, EdemaTek™, Dematek™, Tribute®, and JoVi Pak™.

JoVi Pak is shown here to represent this category of items used selectively along with lymphedema bandaging techniques. Prefabricated items can save therapists time and can simplify self-management for the patient. Jo Ann Rovig, producer of JoVi Pak, states, "In my own practice I have used JoVi Paks to protect bony prominences. I have found them very helpful in treating breast, chest wall, and female genital lymphedema. They also work well over the anatomical indentations around the ankle and the knee and benefit in the reshaping of the limb toward the end of treatment."

Custom and ready-made items in a variety of sizes and shapes are available. Figure 8.3, on page 156, illustrates the full-length arm liner. The model is applying a short-stretch bandage over the liner.

Overview of leading manufacturers of lymphedema bandage supplies

Lohmann-Rauscher	Categories of Bandaging Supplies	BSN-Jobst
tg stockinette	Tubular bandage	Tricofix®
Mollelast®	Elastic gauze—fingers/toes	Elastomull®
Cellona®	Padding	Artiflex®
Rosidal® K	Short-stretch bandages	Comprilan®
Idealbinde®		Isoband®
Komprex®	High density foam	

FIGURE 8-2 Examples of Lymphedema Bandaging Supplies Manufactured by BSN-Jobst

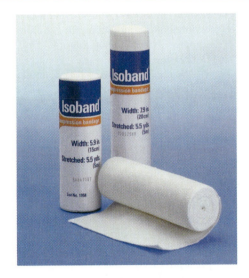

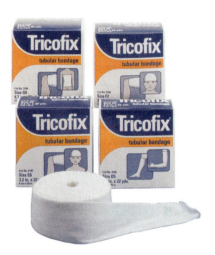

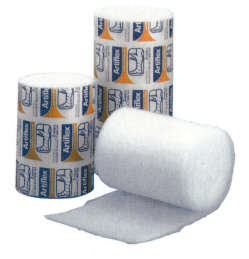

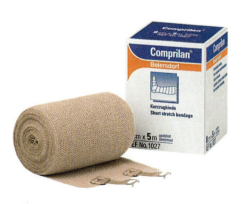

(Courtesy of BSN-Jobst, Inc.)

Recommended Reading

APTA. *Guide to Physical Therapist Practice. Phys Ther.* 2001;8(1):21–746. pp 583.

Aitken RJ, Gaze MN, Rodger A, et al. Arm morbidity within a trial of mastectomy and either nodal sample with selective radiotherapy or axillary clearance. *Br J Surg.* 1989;76: 569–71.

Andersson HC, Parry DM, Mulvihill JJ. Lymphangiosarcoma in late-onset hereditary lymphedema: Case report and nosological implications. *Am J Med Genetics.* 1995; 56: 72–75.

Antony J, Reddy PS. An unusual presentation of carcinoma of the prostate. *J Urology.* 1986; 135:595.

Augustine E. Historical review of external compression for lymphedema management summary of presentation at CSM Boston, MA, February 1998. *Rehab Oncol.* 1998; 16(2): 17–205.

Augustine E, Corn M, Danoff J. Lymphedema management training for physical therapy students in the United States. *Cancer.* 1998; 83 (S12B): 2869–73.

Avrahami R, Haddad M, Zelikovski A. Combined surgical correction of bilateral congenital lower limb lymphedema with associated anomalies. *Lymphology.* 1998; 31:65–67.

Badger CM, Peacock JL, Mortimer PS. A randomized, controlled, parallel-group clinical trial comparing multilayer bandaging followed by hosiery versus hosiery alone in the treatment of patients with lymphedema of the limb. *Cancer.* 2000;88(12):2832–37.

Balzarini A, Pirovano C, Diazzi G, et al. Ultrasound therapy of chronic arm lymphedema after surgical treatment of breast cancer. *Lymphology.* 1993;26:128–34.

Beigel Y, Zelikovski A, Ekstein J, et al. Chylous ascites as a presenting sign of prostatic adenocarcinoma. *Lymphology.* 1990;23: 183–86.

Bertilli G, Venturini M, Forno G, et al. An analysis of prognostic factors in response to conservative treatment of postmastectomy lymphedema. *Surg, GYN &OB.* 1992;175: 455–60.

Bognar J, Nagy P, Kadar E, Bajtal A, Mayer A, Daroczy J, Jaakab F. The current surgical treatment of primary malignant melanoma of the skin. *Acta Chir Hung.* 1997;36:37–38.

Boileau MA, Dowling RA, Gonzales M, et al. Interstitial gold and external beam irradiation for prostate cancer. *J Urolo.* 1988;139:985–88.

Bollinger A, Partsch H, Wolfe JHN, eds. *The Initial Lymphatics;* New Methods and Findings. New York, NY: Thieme-Stratton Inc; 1985.

Borg GA. Psychophyscal bases of perceived exertion. *Med Sci Sports Exerc.* 1982;14(5): 377–81.

Boris M, Weindorf S, Lasinski B. Persistence of lymphedema reduction after noninvasive complex lymphedema therapy. *Oncology.* 1997;11(1):99–109.

Boris M, Weindorf S, Lasinski B. Lymphedema reduction by noninvasive complex lymphedema therapy. *Oncology.* 1994;8(9):95–106.

Bourgeois P, Leduc O, Leduc A. Imaging techniques in the management and prevention of posttherapeutic upper limb edemas. *Cancer.* 1998;83(S12B):2805–13.

Brennan MF. Lymphedema following the surgical treatment of breast cancer: A review of pathophysiology and treatment. *J Pain Symptom Manage.* 1992;7:110–16.

Brennan MJ. Lymphedema following the surgical treatment of breast cancer: A review of pathophysiology and treatment. *Journal of Pain and Symptom Management.* 1992;7(2): 110–16.

Brennan MJ, Depompolo RW, Garden FH. Focused review: Postmastectomy lymphedema. *Arch Phys Med Rehabil* 1996;77: S74–80.

Brennan MJ, Miller LT. Overview of treatment options and review of the current role and use of compression garments, intermittent pumps, and exercise in the management of lymphedema. *Cancer.* 1998;83(S12B):2821–27.

Brorson H, Svensson H. Complete reduction of lymphedema of the arm by liposuction after breast cancer. *Scand J Plast Reconstr Surg.* 1997;31:137–43.

———. Liposuction combined with controlled compression therapy reduces arm lymphedema more effectively than controlled compression therapy alone. *Plastic and Reconstruct Surg.* 1998;102(4):1058–67.

Bull RH, Gane JN, Evans JEC, et al. Abnormal lymph drainage in patients with chronic venous leg ulcers. *J Am Academy Dermat.* 1993;28(4):585–90.

Bunce IH, Mirolo BR, Hennessy JM, et al. Postmastectomy lymphoedema treatment and measurement. *Med J of Australia.* 1994;161: 125–28.

Burgos A, Alcaide A, Alcoba C, et al. Comparative study of the clinical efficacy of two different coumarin dosages in the management of arm lymphedema after treatment for breast cancer. *Lymphology.* 1999; 32:3–10.

Campisi C, Boccarido F. Frontiers in lymphatic microsurgery. *Microsurg.* 1998;18(8):462–71.

Campisi C, Boccarido F, Alitta P, Tacchella M. Derivative lymphatic microsurger: Indications, techniques, and results. *Microsurg.* 1995;16(7):464–68.

Campisi C. Boccarido F, Tacchella M. Reconstructive microsurgery of lymph vessels: The personal method of lymphatic-venous-lymphatic (LVL) interpositioned grafted shunt. *Microsurgery.* 1995;16(3): 161–66.

Carter BJ. Women's experiences of lymphedema. *Oncol Nurs Forum.* 1997;24(5):875–82.

Casley-Smith JR. The fine structure and functioning of tissue channels and lymphatics. *Lymphology.* 1980;12:177–83.

———. Varying total tissue pressures and the concentration of initial lymphatic lymph. *Microvascular Research.* 1983;25:369–79.

———. Alterations of untreated lymphedema and its grades over time. *Lymphology.* 1995; 28:174–85.

———. Treatment of lymphedema by complex physical therapy, with and without oral and topical benzopyrones: What should therapists and patients expect. *Lymphology.* 1996;29:76–82.

Casley-Smith JR, Boris M, Weindorf S, Lasinski B. Treatment for lymphedema of the arm—the Casley-Smith method: A noninvasive method produces continued reduction. *Cancer.* 1998;83(S12B):2843–60.

Chen HC, O'Brien B, Pribaz JJ, Roberts AHN. The use of tonometry in the assessment of upper extremity lymphedema. *Br J Plast Surg.* 1988;41:399–402.

Clodius L, Deak L, Piller NB. A new instrument for the evaluation of tissue tonicity in lymphedema. *Lymphology.* 1976;9:1–5.

Consensus Document of the International Society of Lymphology Executive Committee. The diagnosis and treatment of peripheral lymphedema. *Lymphology.* 1995; 28:113–17.

Cornish BH et al. Early diagnosis of lymphedema in postsurgery breast cancer patients. *Ann N Y Acad Sci.* 2000;904:571–75.

Coward DD. Lymphedema prevention and management knowledge in women treated for breast cancer. *Onc Nurs Forum.* 1999;26(6): 1047–53.

DeLisa JA. *Rehabilitation Medicine: Principles and Practice.* 2nd ed. Philadelphia: Lippincott 1993. 1087–88.

DeLisa JA, Gans BM, eds. *Rehabilitation Medicine: Principles and Practice.* Philadelphia, PA: Lippincott; 1993, 2nd ed.

Dennis B. Acquired lymphedema: A chart review of nine women's responses to intervention. *Am J Occup Ther.* 1993;47:891–99.

Designing Resistance Training Programs. 2nd ed. Fleck, SJ and Kraemer WJ. eds. *Human Kinetics.* 1997.

Dewar KA, Sarrazin D, Benhamou E, et al. Management of the axilla in conservatively treated breast cancer: 592 patients treated at Institut Gustave-Roussy. *Int J Radiat Oncol Biol Phys.* 1987;13:475–81.

Dini D, Del Mastro L, Gozza A, et al. The role of pneumatic compression in the treatment of postmastectomy lymphedema. A randomized phase III study. *Annals of Oncology.* 1998;9:187–90.

Doublet JD, Gattegno B, Thibault P. Laparoscopic pelvic lymph node dissection for staging of prostatic cancer. *Eur Urol.* 1994; 25:194–98.

Elhay S, Casley-Smith JR. *Microvasc Res.* 1976;12:121–40.

Eliska O, Eliskova M. Are peripheral lymphatics damaged by high pressure manual massage? *Lymphology.* 1995;28:21–30.

Ernster VL, Barclay J, Kerlikowske K, et al. Incidence and treatment of ductal carcinoma in situ of the breast. *JAMA.* 1996;275 (12):913–18.

Evans AL, Brice G, Sotirova V, et al. Mapping of primary congenital lymphedema to the 5q35.3 region. *Am J Hum Genet.* 1999;64: 547–55.

Farncombe M, Daniels G, Cross L. Lymphedema: The seemingly forgotten complication. *J Pain and Symptom Manag.* 1994;9(4):269–76.

Földi E. Massage and damage to lymphatics. *Lymphology.* 1995;28:1–3.

———. The treatment of lymphedema. *Cancer.* 1998;83(S12B):2833–34.

Földi E, Foldi M, Clodius L. The lymphedema chaos: A lancet. *Ann Plast Surg.* 1989;22:505–15.

Földi E, Foldi M, Weissleder H. Conservative treatment of lymphoedema of the limbs. *Angioogy.* 1985;36(3):171–80.

———. Are there enigmas concerning the pathophysiology of lymphedema after breast cancer treatment? *NLN Newsletter.* 1998;10(4):1–4.

Földi M. Treatment of lymphedema. (Editorial) *Lymphology.* 1994;27:1–5.

Franzeck UK, et al. Combined physical therapy for lymphedema evaluated by fluorescence microlymphography and lymph capillary pressure measurements. *J Vasc Res.* 1997;34:306–11.

Franzeck UK, Spiegel I, Fischer M, et al. Combined physical therapy for lymphedema evaluated by fluorescence microlymphography and lymph capillary pressure measurements. *J Vasc Research.* 1997;34:306–11.

Ganz PA. Quality of life and cancer rehabilitation. *Rehab Oncology.* 1999;17(3):9–11.

Gerber LH. A review of measures of lymphedema. *Cancer.* 1998;83(S12B):2803–04.

Getz DH. The primary, secondary, and tertiary nursing interventions of lymphedema. *Cancer Nurs.* 1985;8(3):177–84.

Goltner E, Gass P, Haas JP, Schneider P. The importance of volumetry, lymphscintigraphy and computer tomography in the diagnosis of brachial edema after mastectomy. *Lymphology.* 1988;21:134–43.

Greenlee R, Hoyme H, Witte M, et al. Developmental disorders of the lymphatic system. *Lymphology.* 1993;26:156–68.

Grossman IC, Carpiniello V, Greenberg SH, et al. Staging pelvic lymphadeuectomy for carcinoma of the prostate: Review of 91 cases. *J Urol.* 1980;124:632–34.

Guide to physical therapist practice. *Phys Ther* 1997;77(11):1163–1650.

Guyton AC, Barber BJ. The energetics of lymph formation. *Lymphology.* 1980;13:173–76.

Hills NH, Pflug JJ, Jeyasingh K et al. Prevention of deep vein thrombosis by intermittent pneumatic compression of calf. *Br Med J.* 1972;1:131–35.

Holford CP. Graded compression for preventing deep venous thrombosis. *Br Med J.* 1976;2:969–70.

Holmes BM, Ignoffo RJ, Fore C, et al. *Cancer Practice.* 1998;6(2):73–76.

Hwang JH, et al. Changes in lymphatic function after complex physical therapy for lympedema. *Lymphology.* 1999;32:15–21.

Hwang JH, Kwon JY, Lee KW, et al. Changes in lymphatic function after complex physical therapy for lymphedema. *Lymphology.* 1999;32(1):15–21.

International Classification of Functioning and Disability-Beta 2 Draft, Full Version July 1999, World Health Organization Geneva, Switzerland (ICIDH-2) p 9.

International Classification of Impairments, Disabilities and Handicaps. 1994 World Health Organization, Geneva, Switzerland (ICIDH).

Iturregui-Pagan JR. Surgical treatment of post radiotherapy lymphedema. *Biol Assoc Med P Rico.* 1988;80(4):132–34.

Jacobs LF, Kepics J, Konecne S, et al. Lymphedema: An "orphan" disease. *PT Magazine.* June, 1996:54–61.

Johannson K, Albertsson M, Ingvar C, Ekdahl C. Effects of compression bandaging with or without manual lymph drainage treatment in patients with postoperative arm lymphedema. *Lymphology.* 1999;32:103–10.

Johansson K, Lie E, Ekdahl C, Tindfeldt J. A randomized study comparing manual lymph drainage with sequential pneumatic compression for treatment of postoperative arm lymphedema. *Lymphology.* 1998;31:56–64.

Johnson G, Kupper C, Farrar DJ, Swallow RT. Graded compression stockings: Custom vs. noncustom. *Arch Surg.* 1982;117:69–72.

Johnston MG. The intrinsic lymph pump: Progress and problems. *Lymphology.* 1989;22:116–22.

Karakousis C, Heiser M, Moore R. Lymphedema after groin dissection. *Am J Surg.* 1983;145:205–08.

Kasseroller RG. The Vodder school: The Vodder method. *Cancer.* 1998;83(S12B):2840–42.

Kavoussi LR, Sosa E, Chandhoke P, et al. Complications of laparoscopic pelvic lymph node dissection. *J Urolo*. 1993;149:322–25.

Kerr A. Catching lymphedema 'on tape.' *ADVANCE for Phys Ther &PT Assistants*. November, 1998:31.

Kissin MW, Querci della Rovere G, Easton D, Westbury G. Risk of lymphoedema following the treatment of breast cancer. *Br J Surg*. 1986;73:580–84.

Klein MJ, Alexander MA, Wright JM, Redmond CK, LaGasse AA. Treatment of adult lower extremity lymphedema with the Wright Linear pump: Statistical analysis of a clinical trial. *Arch PM&R*. 1988;69:202–06.

Knight KR, Collopy PA, McCain JJ, et al. Protein metabolism and fibrosis in experimental canine obstructive lymphedema. *J Lab Clin Med*. November, 1987:558–66.

Knight KR, Ritz M, Lepore DA, et al. Autologous lymphocyte therapy for experimental canine lymphoedema: A pilot study. *Aust N Z Surg*. 1994;64:332–37.

Ko D, Lerner R, Klose G, Cosimi AB. Effective treatment of lymphedema of the extremities. *Arch Surg*. 1998;133:452–58.

Larson D, Weinstein M, Goldberg I, et al. Edema of the arm as a function of the extent of axillary surgery in patients with stage I-II carcinoma of the breast treated with primary radiotherapy. *Int J Radiat Oncol Biol Phys*. 1986;12(9):1575–82.

Latchford S, Casley-Smith JR. Estimating limb volumes and alterations in peripheral edema from circumferences measured at different intervals. *Lymphology*. 1997;30:161–64.

Le Postollec M. HCFA agrees to pay for lymphedema treatment. *ADVANCE for Phys Thers & PT Assist*. December, 1998:5–6.

Leduc A, Caplan I, Leduc O. Lymphatic drainage of the upper limb. Substitution lymphatic pathways. *EurJ Lymphology*. 1993;4(13):11–17.

Leduc O, Leduc A, Bourgeois P, Belgrado J. The physical treatment of the upper limb edema. *Cancer*. 1998;83(S12B):2835–39.

Leduc O, Peeters A, Borgeois P. Bandages: Scintigraphic demonstration of its efficacy on colloidal protein reabsorption during muscle activity. *Progress in Lymphology-X11*. 1990 Elsevier Science Publishers.

Lee BY, Trainor FS, Kavner D et al. Noninvasive prevention of thrombosis of deep veins of the thigh using intermittent pneumatic compression. *Surg Gyn & Obst*. 1976;142:705–14.

Leitch AM, Meek AG, Smith RA, et al. Workgroup I: Treatment of the axilla with surgery and radiation—Preoperative and postoperative risk assessment. *Cancer*. 1998;83(S12B):2877–79.

Lerner R. Complete decongestive physiotherapy and the Lerner Lymphedema Services Academy of Lymphatic Studies. Supplement to *Cancer*. 1998;83(S12B):2861–63.

————. What's new in lymphedema therapy in America? *International Journal of Angiology*. 1998;7:191–196.

Lerner R, Requena R. Upper extremity lymphedema secondary to mammary cancer treatment. *Am J Clin Oncol*. 1986;9(6):481–87.

Lewis CB, Botomley JM. *Geriatric Physical Therapy—A clinical approach*. Norwalk, CT: Appleton & Lange. 1994.

Lieskovsky G, Skinner DG, Weisenburger T. Pelvic lymphadeuectomy in the management of carcinoma of the prostate. *J Urol*. 1980;124:635–38.

Loprinzi CL, Kuger JW, Sloan JA, et al. Lack of effect of coumarin in women with lymphedema after treatment for breast cancer. *N Engl J Med*. 1999;340:346–50.

Louton RB, Terranova WA. The use of suction curettage as adjunct to the management of lymphedema. *Ann Plastic Surg*. 1989;22(4):354–57.

Mark B. Lymphedema: Etiology and management techniques. *J OB/GYN PT*. 1994;18(2):5–6.

Markowski J, Wilcox JP, Helm PA. Lymphedema incidence after specific postmastectomy therapy. *Arch Phys Med Rehabil*. 1981;62:449–52.

Martimbeau P, Kjorstad K, Kolstad P. Stage 1B carcinoma of the cervix, the Norwegian Radium Hospital, 1968–1970. Results of treatment and major complications. *Am J Obstet Gynecol*. 1978;131:389–94.

Martini FH. *Fundamentals of Anatomy and Physiology* 4th ed. Prentice Hall 1989. pp 769–813.

McGarvey C. Pneumatic compression devices for lymphedema. *Rehab Onc*. 1998;16(3):28.

McIvor J, Tyagi G. Lymphatic hypoplasia without lymphoedema. *Clin Radiol.* 1984;35: 503–05.

Meek AG. Breast radiotherapy and lymphedema. *Cancer.* 1998;83(S12B):2788–97.

Megens A, Harris SR. Physical therapist management of lymphedema following treatment for breast cancer: A critical review of its effectiveness. *Phys Ther.* 1998;78(12):1302–11.

Miller GE, Seale J. Lymphatic clearance during compressive loading. *Lymphology.* 1981;14: 161–66.

Miller LT. The use of resistive and aerobic exercise in the management of breast cancer lymphedema. *Rehab Onc.* 1998;16(3):11–14.

Miller TA. Surgical approach to lymphedema of the arm after mastectomy. *Am J Surg.* 1984;148(1):152–56.

Morgan RG, Casley-Smith JR, Mason MR, Casley-Smith JR. Complex physical therapy for the lymphoedematous arm. *J Hand Surg (Br).* 1992;17B:437–41.

Morrison WA. Lymphedema: The role of microlymphatic surgery. *Perspect Plastic Surg.* 1990;4(1):27–47.

Mortimer PS. The pathophysiology of lymphedema. *Cancer.* 1998;83(S12B):2798–2802.

———. Implications of the lymphatic system in CVI-Associated edema. *Angiology* 2000; 51:3–7.

Mortimer PS, et al. The measurement of skin lymph flow by isotope clearance-reliability, reproductibility, injection dynamics and the effect of massage. *J Invest Dermatol.* 1990; 95(6):677–82.

Mutoh S, Aikou I, Soejima K, et al. Local control of prostate cancer by intraarterial infusion chemotherapy facilitated by the use of antiotension II. *Urol Int.* 1992;48:175–80.

Nagi S. 1969. *Disability and Rehabilitation.* Columbus, OH: Ohio State University Press.

Nava VM, Lawrence WT. Liposuction on a lymphedematous arm. *Ann Plastic Surg.* 1988; 21(4):366–68.

Nishi M, Uchino S, Yabuki S, eds. Hemodynamic effects of pressotherapy. *Progress in Lymphology—XII.* Elsevier Science Publishers B.V. 1990.

O'Brien BM, Khazanchi RK, Kumar PAV, et al. Liposuction in the treatment of lymphoedema: A preliminary report. *Br J Plastic Surg.* 1989;42:530–33.

Olszewski W. On the pathomechanism of development of postsurgical lymphedema. *Lymphology.* 1973;6:35–51.

Olszewski WL, Engeset A. Intrinsic contractility of prenodal lymph vessels and lymph flow in human leg. *Am J Physiol.* 1980;239(6): H775–83.

Pappas CJ, O'Donnell TF. Long-term results of compression treatment for lymphedema. *J Vasc Surg.* 1992;16:555–64.

Passik SD, McDonald MV. Psychosocial aspects of upper extremity lymphedema in women treated for breast carcinoma. *Cancer.* 1998;83(S12B):2817–20.

Petereit DG, Mehta MP, Buchler DA, Kinsella T. A retrospective review of nodal treatment for vulvar cancer. *Am J Clin Oncol.* 1993;16(1):38–42.

Petrek JA. News from MSKCC: *Cancer News:* June 1998. *www.Mskcc.org.*

Petrek JA, Heelan M. Incidence of breast carcinoma-related lymphedema. *Cancer.* 1998;83(S12B):2776–81.

Petrek JA, Pressman PI, Smith RA. Lymphedema: Current issues in research and management. *CA Cancer J Clin.* 2000;50: 292–307.

Pezner RD, Patterson MP, Hill LR, et al. Arm lymphedema in patients treated conservatively for breast cancer: Relationship to patient age and axillary node dissection technique. *J Radiat Oncol Biol Phys.* 1986;12(12):2079–83.

Pilepich MV, Asbell SO, Mulholland GS, Pajak T. Surgical staging in carcinoma of the prostate: The RTOG experience. *The Prostate.* 1984;5:471–76.

Pilepich MV, Krall J, George FW, et al. Treatment-related morbidity in phase III RTOG studies of extended-field irradiation of carcinoma of the prostate. *Int J Radiation Oncology Biol Phys.* 1984;10:1861–67.

Piller NB. Conservative treatment of acute and chronic lymphoedema with benzo-pyrones. *Lymphology.* 1976;9:132–37.

———. Lymphoedema, macrophages and benzopyrones. *Lymphology.* 1980;13:109–19.

Piller NB, Clodius L. The use of a tissue tonometer as a diagnostic aid in extremity lymphoedema: A determination of its conservative treatment with benzo-pyrones. *Lymphology.* 1976;9:127–32.

Piller NB, Thelander A. Treatment of chronic postmastectomy lymphedema with low level laser therapy: A 2.5 year follow-up. *Lymphology*. 1998;31:74–86.

Pressman PI. Surgical treatment and lymphedema. *Cancer*. 1998;83(S12B):2782–82.

Price J, Putrell JR. Prevention and treatment of lymphedema after breast cancer. *Am J Nurs*. 1997;97(9):34–37.

Raines JK, O'Donnell TF, Kalisher L, Darling RC. Selection of patients with lymphedema for compression therapy. *Am J Surg*. 1977; 133:430–37.

Rainwater LM, Zincke H. Radical prostatectomy after radiation therapy for cancer of the prostate: Feasibility and prognosis. *J Urolo*. 1988;140:1455–59.

Ramelet AA. Pharmacologic aspects of a phlebotropic drug in CVI-associated edema. *Angiology*. 2000;51:19–23.

Richmand DM, O'Donnell TF, Zelikovski A. Sequential pneumatic compression for lymphedema: A controlled trial. *Arch Surg*. 1985;120:1116–19.

Rinehart-Ayres ME. Conservative approaches to lymphedema treatment. *Cancer*. 1998;83(S12B):2828–32.

Rockson, et al. Workgroup III: Diagnosis and management of lymphedema. *Cancer* (Supplement) 1998;83(12)2882–85.

Rockson SG, Miller LT, Senie R, et al. Workgroup III: Diagnosis and management of lymphedema. *Cancer* (Supplement). 1998;83(S12B):2882–85.

Rudkin G, Miller T. Lipedema: A clinical entity distinct from lymphedema. *Plastic and Reconstructive Surgery*. 1994;91(6):841–47.

Runowicz CD. Lymphedema: Patient and provider education: Current status and future trends. *Cancer*. 1998;83(S12B): 2874–76.

Runowicz CD, Passik SD, Hann D, et al. Workgroup II: Patient education—pre- and posttreatment. *Cancer*. 1998;83(S12B): 2880–81.

Ryan TJ, Curri SB. The microcirculation of fat in man: The importance of the regulation of blood flow. *Clinics in Dermaologyt*. 1989; 7(4):25–36.

Sabris S, Roberts V, Cotton LT. Prevention of early postoperative deep vein thrombosis by intermittent compression of the leg during surgery. *Br Med J*. 1971;4:394–96.

Salner AL. Lymphedema following prostatectomy and radiation therapy. *Cancer Pract*. 1998;6(2):73–76.

Savage RC. The surgical management of lymphedema. *Surg Gynecol Obstet*. 1985;160: 283–90.

Schenkman M, et al. Multisystem model for management of neurologically impaired adults—An update and illustrative case. *Neurology Report*. 1999;23(4):145–57.

Schmid-Schonbein GW. Microlymphatics and lymph flow. *Physiol Rev*. 1990;70(4): 987–1028.

Servelle M. Surgical treatment of lymphedema: A report on 652 cases. *Surgery*. April, 1987:485–95.

Sewell RA, Braren V, Wilson SK, Rhamy RK. Extended biopsy follow-up after full course radiation for resectable prostatic carcinoma. *J Urol*. 1975;113:371–73.

Shea B, Kleban R, Knauer CJ. Breast cancer rehabilitation. *Seminars Surg Oncol*. 1991; 7:326–30.

Shipley WU, Kopelson G, Novack DH, et al. Preoperative irradiation, lymphadenectomy and 125iodine implant for patients with localized prostatic carcinoma: A correlation of implant dosimetry with clinical results. *J Urol*. 1980;124:639–42.

Sigel B, Edelstein A, Savitch L, et al. Types of compression for reducing venous stasis. *Arch Surg*. 1975;110:171–75.

Smith J. The practice of venepuncture in lymphoedema. *Eur J Cancer Care*. 1998;7:97–98.

Smith R. Introduction. *Cancer*. 1998;83(S12B): 2775.

Smith T. Breast cancer update—1999. *Rehab Oncol*. 1999;17(1):12–16.

Sordillo PP, Chapman R, Hajdu SI, et al. Lymphangiosarcoma. *Cancer*. 1981;48(7): 1674–79.

Stemmer R, Marescaux J, Furderer C. Compression therapy of the lower extremities particularly with compression stockings. *Hautarzt (Dermatologist)*. 1980;31:355–65. Article in German.

Svensson WE, Mortimer PS, Tohno E, Cosgrove DO. Increased arterial inflow demonstrated by Doppler ultrasound in arm swelling following breast cancer treatment. *Eur J Cancer*. 1994;30A(5):661–64.

Swedborg I, Norrefalk J, Piller NB, Asard C. Lymphoedema post-mastectomy: Is elevation alone an effective treatment? *Scand J Rehab Med*. 1993;25:79–82.

Swirsky J, Nannery DS. *Coping with Lymphedema*. 1998. Garden City Park, NY: Avery Publishing Group.

Szuba A, Rockson SG. Lymphedema: Anatomy, physiology and pathogenesis. *Vasc Med*. 1997:2:321–26.

———. Lymphedema: Classification, diagnosis and therapy. *Vasc Med*. 1998;3:145–56.

Tadych K, Donegan WL. Postmastectomy seromas and wound drainage. *Surg Gynecol Obstet*. 1987;165:483–87.

Tasmuth T, von Smitten K, Hietanen P, et al. Pain and other symptoms after different treatment modalities of breast cancer. *Ann Oncol*. 1995:453–59.

Thiadens SRJ. Current status of education and treatment resources for lymphedema. *Cancer*. 1998;83(S12B):2864–68.

Tiedjen KU, Kluken N. Isotope lymphographic research in connection with postthrombotic and lymphatic oedema under therapy with diuretics. *Progress in Lymphology*. 1981; 282–85.

Tobin MB, Lacey HJ, Meyer L, Mortimer PS. The psychological morbidity of breast cancer—related to breast cancer. *Cancer*. 1993;72(11):3248–52.

Trattner A, Shamai-Lubovitz O, Segal R, Zelikovski A. Stewart-Treves angiosarcoma of arm and ipsilateral breast in post-traumatic lymphedema. *Lymphology*. 1996;29:57–59.

Tsyb AF, Bardychev MS, Guseva LI. Secondary limb edemas following irradiation. *Lymphology*. 1981;14:127–32.

Tumolo J. Treating lymphedema with CDP. *ADVANCE for Physical Therapists and PT Assistants*. May 15, 1999. 43–45.

Tunkel RS, Cohen S. Lymphedema management. *Rehabilitation Oncology*. 2000;18(1).

Tunkel RS, Lachmann E. Lymphedema of the limb: An overview of treatment options. *Postgraduate Medicine*. 1998;104(4): 131–44.

Velanovich V, Szymanski W. Quality of life of breast cancer patients with lymphedema. *Am J Surgery*. 1999;177:184–88.

Verbrugge LM, Jette AM. The disablement process. *Soc Sci Med*. 1994 Jan;38(1):1–14

Walley DR, Augustine E, Saslow D, et al. Workgroup IV: Lymphedema treatment resources—professional education and availability of patient services. *Cancer*. 1998;83(S12B):2886–87.

Weiss JM. Treatment of leg edema and wounds in a patient with severe musculoskeletal injuries. *Phys Ther*. 1998;78(10):1104–13.

Weissleder H, Schuchhardt C. *Lymphedema, Diagnosis and Therapy*, 2d ed. 1997. Bonn, Germany: Kagerer Kommunication.

Weissleder H, Weissleder R. Lymphedema: Evaluation of qualitative and quantitative lymphoscintigraphy in 238 patients. *Radiology*. 1988; 167:729–35.

Weissleder R, Thrall JH. The lymphatic system: Diagnostic imaging studies. *Radiology*. 1989;172:315–17.

Werner GT, Scheck R, Kaiserling E. Magnetic resonance imaging of peripheral lymphedema. *Lymphology*. 1998;31:34–36.

Werngren-Elgstrom M, Lidman D. Lymphoedema of the lower extremities after surgeries and radiotherapy for cancer of the cervix. *Scand J Plast Reconstr Hand Surg*. 1994; 28:289–93.

Whitman M, McDaniel RW. Preventing lymphedema: An unwelcome sequel to breast cancer. *Nursing*. 1993:36–39.

Wittlinger H. *Textbook of Dr. Vodder's Manual Lymphatic Drainage* II. 1989. Heidelberg, Germany: Karl R. Hang Publishers.

INDEX